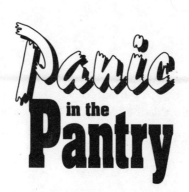

Consumer Health Library®
Series Editor: Stephen Barrett, M.D.
Technical Editor: Manfred Kroger, Ph.D.

Other titles in this series:

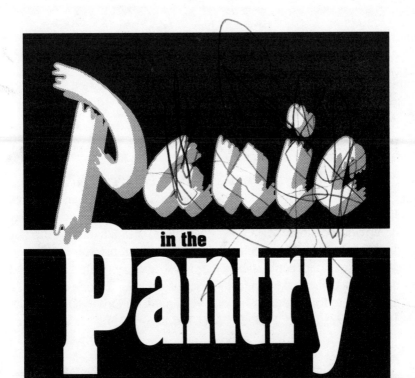

Panic

in the

Pantry

Facts & Fallacies about the Food You Buy

**Elizabeth M. Whelan, Sc.D., M.P.H.
and Fredrick J. Stare, M.D., Ph.D.**

edited by Stephen Barrett, M.D.

Prometheus Books • Buffalo, New York

Published 1992 by Prometheus Books

96   95   94   93   92   5   4   3   2   1

Library of Congress Cataloging-in-Publication Data

Whelan, Elizabeth M.
    Panic in the pantry : facts and fallacies about the food
you buy / by Elizabeth M. Whelan and Fredrick J. Stare.
       p.   cm.
    Originally published: New York : Atheneum, 1975
    Includes bibliographical references (p.   ) and index.
    ISBN 0-87975-732-9
    1. Food additives. 2. Natural foods. I. Stare, Fredrick J.
(Fredrick John), 1910–   . II. Title
TX 553.A3W44 1992
613.2--dc20
                                     92-7986
                                        CIP

Printed in Canada on acid-free paper.

Contents

Preface

When the first edition of *Panic in the Pantry* was published in 1975, we were very gratified by the public acceptance it received. In addition to going through several printings, our original book was translated into Japanese and French.

We would like to be able to say that in the ensuing years the American public has become more realistic about the safety and quality of its food supply. Unfortunately, this isn't so. People still cringe at the long names of chemicals that are purposefully added or just happen to end up in our food. At times this fear is understandable—but it is not scientifically justified.

Americans are tired of being told that they are being poisoned by everything around them. And yet many continue to react to whatever they hear or read—whether the source is reliable or not. Even though we have the safest food supply in the world, repeated claims that our food supply is tainted have caused increasing fearfulness. We have been told that widely used food colors are harmful even though there have been no demonstrable ill effects. Hot dogs, Chinese food, breakfast cereals, coffee, and many other popular items have also been accused of harboring dangerous chemicals. Each new criticism not only arouses concern about the item under attack, but also contributes to general distrust of our food supply.

The worst "panic" in recent years has probably been the Alar scare of 1989. The media circus that led to Alar's removal from the marketplace caused serious harm to apple growers as well as American consumers—despite the fact that human health was never even remotely threatened.

Panic in the Pantry was written to help you become fully aware of the *real* facts behind news about the safety of our food supply. In this book we examine the power wielded by health food faddists who band together and exert political pressure to protect their profitable ventures. We explain why the concept of "relative risk" should be used to place information about food additives and preservatives into proper perspective. We show why the Delaney Clause—a law intended to protect us from cancer-causing chemicals in our food—cannot fulfill the noble purpose for which it was drafted and therefore should be repealed. We evaluate the research behind the banning of cyclamates and the attacks on saccharin and aspartame that have left many Americans wondering whether they are doomed to either be chubby or develop cancer. And our discussion of California's Proposition 65 provides insight into the chaos that can result when fearmongers are able to secure legislation based on panic about our food supply.

Since *Panic in the Pantry* first hit bookstore shelves around the world, some misinformation has been cleared up. But, as we demonstrate in this update, it appears to have been replaced by even more.

Elizabeth M. Whelan, Sc.D., M.P.H.
Fredrick J. Stare, M.D., Ph.D.

About the Authors

• Elizabeth M. Whelan, Sc.D., M.P.H., holds advanced degrees in epidemiology and public health from the Yale University School of Medicine and the Harvard School of Public Health. She is cofounder and president of the American Council on Science and Health (ACSH) and publisher of the council's quarterly magazine *Priorities: For Long Life and Good Health*. She has been a member of the U.S. Department of Agriculture's advisory committee on meat and poultry inspection, the Environmental Protection Agency's advisory committee on pesticides and toxics, and the American Cancer Society's national committee on cancer prevention and detection. She has moderated the nationally syndicated radio program "Healthline" and is a contributing editor to *American Baby*, *Mirabella*, and *Private Practice*. In 1986 she won the American Medical Writer's Association Walter Alvarez Award for excellence in medical communication. She is author or coauthor of twenty-three books, including: *Toxic Terror: The Truth Behind the Cancer Scare; Preventing Cancer; A Baby? Maybe;* and *A Smoking Gun: How the Cigarette Industry Gets Away with Murder*.

• Fredrick J. Stare, M.D., Ph.D., is Professor Emeritus of Nutrition and founder of Harvard University's Department of Nutrition. He is also cofounder and a board member of the American Council on Science and Health. He was a member of the Food and Nutrition Board of the National Research Council for many years, and has served as consultant to numerous voluntary and governmental agencies, food companies and trade associations. One of the world's most prominent nutritionists, he has received awards from seven major professional societies.

Dr. Stare is author or coauthor of seventeen books, more than four hundred research and review articles in peer-reviewed scientific journals, and many other articles in lay publications. He was, for twenty-five years, editor of the prestigious journal *Nutrition Reviews*. He wrote a nationally syndicated newspaper column for nearly forty years and has also moderated a syndicated radio program. His books include *Eating for Good Health; Living Nutrition; Eat OK—Feel OK;* and three books written with Dr. Whelan: *Balanced Nutrition: Beyond the Cholesterol Scare; The Harvard Square Diet;* and *The 100% Natural, Purely Organic, Cholesterol-Free, Megavitamin, Low-Carbohydrate Nutrition Hoax.* His most recent books are *Your Guide to Good Nutrition* and an autobiography titled *Adventures in Nutrition.*

About the Editor

• Stephen Barrett, M.D., who practices psychiatry in Allentown, Pennsylvania, is a nationally renowned author, editor, and consumer advocate. An expert in medical communications, he edits *Nutrition Forum Newsletter* and is medical editor of Prometheus Books. He is a board member of the National Council Against Health Fraud and chairs the council's Task Force on Victim Redress. His thirty-one books include: *The Health Robbers; Vitamins and "Health" Foods: The Great American Hustle; Health Schemes, Scams, and Frauds;* and the college textbook *Consumer Health: A Guide to Intelligent Decisions.* In 1984 he won the FDA Commissioner's Special Citation Award for Public Service in fighting nutrition quackery. In 1987 he began teaching health education at The Pennsylvania State University.

Acknowledgements

The authors are grateful to the following individuals for their many helpful suggestions during the preparation of the manuscript:

Editorial consultants
Associate editor for revision Mary Carole McMann, M.P.H., R.D.
                               Houston, Texas
Project manager   Mary A. Read, Prometheus Books
Technical editor   Manfred Kroger, Ph..D.
                               Professor of Food Science
                               The Pennsylvania State University

Scientific consultants
Lisa T. Harris, R.D.   Rialto, California
William T. Jarvis, Ph.D.   Professor of Public Health
                               and Preventive Medicine
                               Loma Linda University
                               School of Medicine
Patricia Kuntze   FDA Office of Consumer Affairs
Marilyn G. Stephenson,   Assistant to the Director
    M.S., R.D.   FDA Office of Nutrition and
                               Food Sciences

Library consultants   FDA Library, Rockville, Md.
                               Jesse H. Jones Library
                               Texas Medical Center
                               University of Oklahoma
                               Health Sciences Center Library
                               Oklahoma County Public Libraries

1

Fear of Eating

Beautiful Soup, so rich and green,
Waiting in a hot tureen!
Who for such dainties would not stoop?
Soup of the evening, beautiful Soup!
Soup of the evening, beautiful Soup!

—Lewis Carroll
Alice in Wonderland

A Classic Case of Panic

In February 1989, Americans tuned to CBS-TV's "60 Minutes" were shocked to hear Ed Bradley declare that "the most potent cancer-causing agent in our food supply is a substance sprayed on apples to keep them on the trees longer and make them look better." Fifty million viewers were told that Alar (chemical name: daminozide) posed an "intolerable" cancer risk, particularly for children who consume large quantities of apple products relative to their size. To help make its point, CBS showed footage of children in cancer wards.

Mr. Bradley solemnly assured viewers that this story was based on "the most careful study yet on the effect of daminozide

1

and seven other cancer-causing pesticides on the food children eat."

Panic ensued. School systems destroyed apples and apple products. One consumer called the International Apple Institute and asked if it was safe to discard apple juice in the kitchen sink or whether it was necessary to take it to a toxic waste dump. A hysterical parent sent state troopers chasing after her child's school bus to confiscate the forbidden fruit the child was carrying.

"And so began the great apple scare of 1989," wrote *Washington Times* editorialist Kenneth Smith one year later. "The results were not long in coming. Washington's regulatory apparatus cranked up to prevent the looming baby slaughter. The apple industry turned into applesauce as apple prices plummeted and sales fell off. Hysterical parents fretted over lunchbox contents.... School administrators expelled the apple summarily. Taxpayers got stuck with the bill for apple leftovers."

Today it is clear that the great apple scare was a shrewdly orchestrated media extravaganza, based not on scientifically sound evidence but on a report that the scientific community had rejected.

The Natural Resources Defense Council (NRDC) was behind this atrocity. For many years, this group has argued that our food should have no pesticide residues whatsoever. Never mind that the amounts of such residues are minuscule and that our government has set ultrasafe tolerance levels and tests our food supply to ensure that these standards are met.

The only ammunition NRDC had was a single study of mice fed enormous doses of Alar relative to their weight. In this study, one mouse developed one tumor. This study was not repeated with other species. Nor was it peer-reviewed or published in a reputable scientific journal.

The study's weakness did not stop NRDC. They finally

hired media consultant David Fenton to stir things up. Mr. Fenton later said about his efforts:

> Our goal was to create so many repetitions of NRDC's message that average American consumers (not just the policy elite in Washington) could not avoid hearing it—from many different media outlets within a short period of time. The idea was for the "story" to achieve a life of its own, and continue for weeks and months to affect policy and consumer habits.

To bolster his campaign, Fenton enlisted the help of actress Meryl Streep, who, with broadcaster Tom Brokaw's wife, formed "Mothers and Others for Pesticide Limits." Suddenly, Streep became not only the spokesperson for NRDC but a widely quoted expert on food safety.

Fenton struck a deal with CBS whereby the network would present the results of the NRDC study so long as CBS was given exclusive access to it. His plan worked exceedingly well. The "60 Minutes" exclusive was followed by a news conference the next day and with numerous talk show appearances and magazine cover stories in the weeks that followed.

It was virtually impossible to miss the alarming news. But Americans who threw out their apples and apple products apparently heard little or nothing about the following:

• The Environmental Protection Agency (EPA) sets tolerance levels on pesticides. Only minuscule amounts of residue are allowed, and the FDA makes sure that these levels are not exceeded. Alar residues were well within the permitted tolerance.

• Other than one high-dosage mouse study, there was no evidence to indicate that Alar posed any health hazard whatever to humans, not even to children who consume relatively large amounts of apples and apple products. The National Cancer Institute had studied the effects of Alar on both mice and rats in 1966 and again in 1978, finding no increases in tumors.

• It was extrapolation, not testing, that led to any concern at all. Further tests that the EPA ordered in 1986 also failed to produce tumors. The agency then quadrupled dosages until 80 percent of the mice were dying from toxicity alone—not cancer. At these excessive doses, just one mouse developed a tumor. Without reason, the EPA extrapolated from this one lonely tumor that the risk to the population from Alar is forty-five cancers per million people.

• EPA's own Scientific Advisory Panel on Alar had repeatedly rejected pleas to ban Alar because they thought the rodent data were inadequate. In other words, the EPA's experts did not conclude that Alar posed a threat to human health.

• The doses used in the mouse study were exceedingly large. To even come close to an equivalent dosage, a child would have to drink 19,000 quarts of apple juice per day throughout life. Put another way, the mice received a dose 22,000 times the maximum exposure of children, or 266,000 times *normal* ingestion. Further, this toxicity assessment was downgraded in late 1991, when EPA studies revealed that Alar and its byproduct UDMH are really only half as potent as the agency estimated during the Alar crisis in 1989. That means that the EPA is now saying their risk estimates are based on doses greater than half a million times normal human ingestion.

• In 1989, the British government concluded that there "was no risk to health" from Alar or UDMH. The chairman of the group appointed to advise the British Parliament said that its view differed from that of the EPA because "we tend to be a bit more cautious" about science. "We don't always make the assumption that the animal data are transferable to man," he said, adding that high-dose exposure of animals is not directly relevant to low-dose human exposure.

• Other international views echo those of the British. A United Nations panel concluded in 1989 that Alar was "not oncogenic in mice" and that UDMH raised no special concern. The group, which included seven members from the World Health Organization (WHO) and seven from the Food and Agriculture Organization (FAO), was confident of its opinion and set a high tolerance for Alar residues in food.

• Finally, only 15 percent of America's apple trees were sprayed with Alar.

NRDC's disgraceful activities caused the apple industry to suffer severe economic losses. The Apple Institute estimated that apple growers lost $250 million, including $40 million in the state of Washington. Many apple growers lost their businesses, some of which had been in the family for generations. Apple processors lost an estimated $125 million.

Apple growers from Yakima County in the state of Washington have filed a $200 million suit against NRDC, Fenton Communications, and "60 Minutes" for causing such devastating economic losses. The EPA's downgrading of Alar's toxicity is expected to be important evidence in the case.

Gary Flamm, a former Food and Drug Administration (FDA) staffer, has summed up the feelings of scientists who were offended by the environmentalists responsible for the Alar fiasco:

> One has to conclude the publicity [Alar] got really had nothing to do with the science. . . . [Apple growers were] severely injured, and we are not talking about truth, justice, and mercy prevailing. My own feeling is that

scientists who sit by and watch [such] things happen [without protesting are] no different from scientists who fudge data.

Perhaps the scientific truth can be summed up best by quotes from the press conference held by the American Council on Science and Health on the third anniversary of the Great Alar Scare:

A chemical is currently tested for cancer by feeding massive doses to laboratory animals. These doses are much higher, sometimes hundreds of thousands of times higher, than humans will be exposed to. . . . The calculated cancer risk values are theoretically worst-case numbers, which bear no absolutely relationship to real risk. Unfortunately, these numbers take on a life of their own and are used to convince people that pesticides in food are dangerous to their health.

> Joseph D. Rosen, Ph.D.
> Cook College
> Rutgers University

As a pediatric surgeon, as well as the nation's former Surgeon General, I care deeply about the health of children, and if Alar ever posed a health hazard I would have said so then and would say so now. But the truth is that Alar never did pose a health hazard. The American food supply is not only the most abundant in the world, but it is also the safest. Paradoxically—it has achieved that position in the world market just because of chemicals like Alar that have made it possible.

> C. Everett Koop, M.D.
> Chairman
> National Safe Kids Campaign

There are two kinds of environmentalists . . . scientific environmentalists who rely on science . . . and others who rely upon ideology rather than science. It's imperative that the media insist upon outstanding science and nothing less as the basis for decision-making in environmental protection. Those who exaggerate the effects of environmental pollutants do not act in the interest of human health and environmental protection. . . . The Alar controversy is a classic case of poor science poorly applied to a societal decision, resulting in a poor final decision.

> Alan A. Moghissi, Ph.D.
> University of Maryland

When used in the approved regulated fashion, as it was, Alar does not pose a risk to the public's health. In matters of health, good science, not misplaced fears, must drive public policy.

> Ralph R. Reed, M.D.
> Senior Medical Advisor
> American Medical Association

The risk of eating an apple treated with Alar is less than the risk of eating a peanut butter sandwich or a well done hamburger.

> Richard Adamson
> National Cancer Institute

Maintaining Your Perspective

The Alar apple scare illustrates how unfounded fears about our food supply can have far-reaching effects. Consumers wishing to avoid "panic in the pantry" should keep the following in mind:

1. Peer-reviewed, mainstream science, the type worthy of reporting to readers or viewers, does not depend upon media manipulations, exclusive agreements, press releases, or Hollywood personalities to gain public acceptance. Nor would it utilize a "left-wing legal activist group," as the *Wall Street Journal* described the NRDC. Solid science is found in reputable journals, where it undergoes peer review prior to publication. Such publication does not guarantee 100 percent accuracy or that future findings will not change, but only that it represents sound science at the time. The fact that peer-reviewed publication is integral to the growth of science is often overlooked by journalists, consumers, and some consumer advocates.

2. Check with other reliable sources at colleges and universities. Don't rely on activists, government regulators, or industry spokespersons to provide objectivity. If you want scientific information, seek the opinions of scientists. They have the expertise.

3. If a purported scientific topic requires a publicity blitz from "60 Minutes," "Donahue," "20/20," or a partisan political group such as the NRDC to gain public attention, beware! The question is not whether the press should have done a better job in presenting NRDC's "Intolerable Risk" study, but whether the media should have reported this study at all.

Panic in the Pantry Is Not New

Unwarranted food scares are not a new phenomenon. During the 1960s Americans went without cranberries for their holiday dinners because of falsely and prematurely reported studies—studies that later were proved wrong. Mushrooms were similarly banished from the grocery cart and subsequently returned.

Events like these have caused Americans to become very worried about food safety. Many people turn to the United States government to assuage their food fears. In 1987 alone, the FDA received 34,599 consumer mail inquiries. Here are excerpts from letters received during 1988 about our food supply:

> Wonder if you could tell me if the FDA has obtained reports on the aflatoxin levels of various brands of peanut butter. Is it a risk to consume a half-jar (9 ounces) daily? Thank you very much for your assistance.

* * *

> I recently read that the FDA routinely gives food additive manufacturers undue periods of time to demonstrate that their products are safe for human consumption. Seems you're making guinea pigs of us all.

* * *

> I have just read an article about radiation checks on products, stating that there is a search for possible low-level radiation contamination in some foods and drink. Now what puzzles me is why the FDA is concerned, due to the fact that you allow irradiation of food for longer shelf life. Please, why are you concerned about one and not the other?

* * *

> If what I have been told and read about these (coconut, palm, and palm kernel) oils is true, I would like to know why they are being so widely used and why you haven't taken steps to have them banned. I'm sure safe oils could be used in place of unsafe ones.

Enclosed please find the side panel of a box of . . . cereal and a photocopy of the back of a box of trisodium phosphate. One of the ingredients listed on the cereal box is trisodium phosphate. The warning listed on the box of trisodium phosphate clearly states that it shouldn't be taken internally. I don't understand how this type of ingredient could be allowed into a food product. An explanation would be appreciated.

* * *

I am highly allergic to artificial colorings but also get reactions from a similar chemical to artificial colors. What chemicals are used to make F, D &C (Food, Drug & Cosmetic) artificial colorings used in food—especially yellow #5 and reds?

Thanks very much—
Any help will be appreciated

A Recipe for Fear

What are the roots of such intense and compelling food fears? Looking back in history (as we'll do in chapter 2), we'll see that people have always been concerned about food safety and been plagued by food myths and misconceptions. The ingredients of most food fears are affluence, the scapegoat phenomenon, agricultural naïveté, chemical naïveté, and the political power of antichemical, antibusiness groups.

  Affluence. Food fears can thrive only in a highly affluent society. Most of the world is preoccupied not with traces of pesticides or additives but with getting enough food to live a healthy life. Only where food is abundant can people afford to throw out perfectly wholesome products—and not feel the immediate economic and health effects of such action.

Scapegoat phenomenon. In primitive societies it was common for people to believe in malevolent witchcraft that would relieve them of guilt or complicity in a tragic occurrence. For example, anthropologist Bronislaw Malinkowsky has noted how African mothers ascribed the death of a child to a spell cast on the child's food by a jealous neighbor. Similarly, Americans find it easier to blame outside influences than to examine their own role in disease causation.

During the early part of this century, our government made great strides in doing things to improve public health—through immunizations, chlorination of water, and other measures. Dramatic improvements occurred with little or no individual effort. Today, however, our focus should be on risk factors for chronic diseases such as heart disease and cancer. Nearly 40 percent of cancer deaths in this country (and many more deaths due to heart disease) are caused by cigarette smoking. What causes most of the other 60 percent of cancer deaths is not known. Yet the media and various consumer groups place far more emphasis on "chemicals" in our food supply than they do in attacking the number-one preventable cause of premature death.

Agricultural naïveté. Most Americans have had very little contact with farms and agricultural science. Our urban centers are so far from the farm heartlands of the country that we are removed from the whole process, and perhaps take too much for granted. Perhaps many of us simply assume that God meant our cereal and oranges to be bug-free.

The reality is that humans compete with insects and other life forms for food. Worldwide crop losses have been estimated to be as high as 45 percent. Pesticides of varying toxicity must be used selectively to kill pests such as insects and their larvae, fungi, root worms, slugs, weeds, rats, mice, and other organisms. Pesticides are an indispensable tool in reducing these depredations. It would be a sad state of affairs if we had to experience widespread food spoilage and shortages before Americans once again become grateful that high-tech agricultural chemicals exist.

Chemical naïveté. For most consumers, chemistry, like agriculture, is an unknown—and unfamiliar things often become targets for unrealistic fears of danger. Many Americans have been brainwashed into believing that what is "natural" is safe, and what is synthetic is suspect. In addition, many believe that even minute traces of a potentially dangerous chemical must be removed from foods.

That is neither possible nor necessary. Scientists have long known that natural foods have plentiful supplies of natural toxins (see chapter 4). For example, shrimp and other shellfish contain arsenic; potatoes are a complex mixture of some 150 known chemicals, including solanine, arsenic, tannins, and nitrate; and lima beans contain that classic suicide potion, hydrogen cyanide. Naturally occurring food toxins are present in such large amounts that removing human-made chemicals from food in an effort to make them toxin-free would be like removing a few grains of sand from a beach.

Political power of antichemical groups. The so-called environmental movement can take the major credit for many, if not all, of the food scares during the past few decades and for the banning of certain food chemicals. The Natural Resources Defense Council, which was responsible for the Alar fiasco, has offices in New York, Washington, San Francisco, Denver, and Natick, Massachusetts, and a yearly budget of over $15 million. It has listed its number-one goal as "the protection of human health and the environment" and has designated itself the self-appointed watchdog of the Environmental Protection Agency. As the NRDC's name implies, litigation is its primary tool for developing and implementing federal regulations related to air, food, and water quality. But it never addresses the *proven* causes of premature disease and death.

Another major player in the business of promoting chemical-phobia is the Center for Science in the Public Interest (CSPI), a Washington-based spin-off of the Ralph Nader empire, with a budget exceeding $4 million a year. CSPI seems to have a contempt for chemicals and the industries that make or use them.

CSPI warns its constituency (and, unfortunately, members of the media) of alleged cancer risks posed by food additives and pesticide residues and is a major promoter of "organically grown" foods. But the data it uses to back up its frightening claims are flimsy at best. For example, CSPI's June 1991 *Nutrition Action Healthletter* listed "The Ten Worst Additives," which they excerpted from their new book *Eating Wisely in a Risky World.* The evidence they used to attack such useful and disease-preventing additives as BHA and BHT was sketchy and focused only on studies in laboratory animals.

Groups like NRDC and CSPI claim to be promoting public health. But it seems to us that they are doing just the opposite by distracting attention from the important health threats that our society should be dealing with. Instead of fretting over apples, Americans should do more about cigarette smoking and AIDS. Instead of worrying about chemicals in baby food, parents should see that children are safety-belted when traveling by car, helmeted when riding a bicycle, and protected by a smoke detector at home.

Fifteen years ago, scientist Dr. Bernard L. Oser predicted that our "exaggerated concern for the safety of foods" would "detract attention from real dangers, as has been happening in the use of tobacco and drugs, particularly by the young." His words have been proven true.

The Shift to "Natural" Foods

In their quest for wholesome food, many Americans alarmed by food scares have turned to what they are told is "natural" or "organic." Have you ever stopped to ask what the term "organic" means? Organic, as you'll read in chapter 3, simply means "food that comes from living organisms." Health food enthusiasts, however, use the term to suggest wholesomeness.

As we detail in chapter 4, all that is natural is not better. For one thing, banning all pesticides, herbicides, and preservatives would seriously threaten our food supply and lead to widespread disease and death. Food chemicals are judiciously used not only to improve crop yield and to maintain affordable food prices, but also to protect consumers from potentially fatal foodborne disease. Nobel Prize winner Dr. Norman E. Borlaug said that without pesticides, crop losses would rise to 50 percent and food prices would increase fourfold to fivefold. In the same vein, former Secretary of Agriculture Earl Butz estimated years ago that fifty million people in the U.S. alone would starve if we were to depend solely on organic farming. Food chemicals also eliminate the threat of potentially fatal food infestation.

Panic in the Nursery

Without a doubt, the panic-in-the-pantry phenomenon has gained momentum, enough to carry it right into the nursery. In mid-1991, the makers of Beech-Nut baby foods announced a new product line, "Beech-Nut Special Harvest." You guessed right:

organic baby food. "Special Harvest" products, assures Beech-Nut, are made with fruits, vegetables, and grains grown without synthetic pesticides. The organic choice was initially available only in Chicago, San Francisco, Phoenix, New York, Los Angeles, Pittsburgh, and Philadelphia, because of the limited availability of organic products. In its press release, Beech-Nut said that "many mothers are surprised to learn that the average cost of using organic baby food is only an additional $4.00 per week." Should we be relieved that the amount wasted is "only" $4.00 a week?

Getting the Facts

Everyone who buys food ought to know the facts about the current natural food craze and about the "panic in the pantry" over food additives and chemicals. At least five basic questions should be asked:

1. *Where does our present additive-phobia fit in terms of history?* Is this back-to-nature craze really all that new? Are there examples of past food scares from which we can learn?

2. *What exactly is the current natural-foods movement all about?* Who is "eating natural," what types of products are they buying, and what are some of the problems associated with America's fascination over "Healthfoodland"?

3. *Is there any truth in the assumptions upon which Healthfoodland is built?* If a food is "natural," does this mean that it is free of "chemicals" and full of health-promoting substances?

4. *What are food additives anyway?* What do they do? And most important: Are they safe? Why were some widely used additives banned? What would happen if all additives were eliminated from our food?

5. *How are food additives regulated today?* What problems are associated with food laws in general and the Delaney anticancer clause in particular? How can these laws be changed to allow a more reasonable regulation of our food supply and to promote a return of confidence in the safety of our food supply?

In the pages that follow, we'll answer these questions. Let's begin by looking at some of the historical (and often hysterical) food fads and see how they managed to capture the minds and stomachs of many unsuspecting eaters of their day.

2

Roots of Fear and Faddism:
A History of "Natural" Eating

". . . a bread-and-butterfly. Its wings are thin
    slices of bread and butter, its body is a
    crust, and its head is a lump of sugar."
"And what does *it* live on?"
"Weak tea with cream in it."
A new difficulty came into Alice's head.
"Supposing it couldn't find any?" she sug-
    gested.
"Then it would die."

—Lewis Carroll
Through the Looking Glass

The Bad-Food/Good-Food Concept

Humans have worried about the safety of food since Adam
looked suspiciously at the apple, eons before the Alar hoax.
While the early food fads stemmed mainly from superstition
and ignorance—the British colonists, for example, believed
that if a man ate a potato every day, he wouldn't live out seven
years—many subsequent fads have involved delusions and/or
greed. The progress that brought urbanization and an increasing

17

dependence on purchased foodstuffs spawned many less-than-scrupulous entrepreneurs. The more sensational their product's claim, of course, the brisker the sales.

Whatever their origin, all food fads have two factors in common. First, they have no sound scientific basis. Second, because they play on fear, many people at whom they are directed don't demand scientific proof. Threats of disease and death have always generated enough fear to persuade some individuals to avoid whatever is attacked. If people who fear cancer hear that milk causes cancer, they may quickly decide to shun milk. Fear drains some people of all rational ability to evaluate food-scare statements.

Some fads identify subcultures. All major religions, for instance, have characteristic food laws. Pope Gregory III, for example, ordered his apostle Boniface to forbid all Christian converts from eating horse flesh; this separated them from pagan tribes who ate horse meat in their rites of worship. Buddhists may not kill animals for food because they believe that "not to injure living things is good." Many Jews exclude pork and shellfish from their diet and avoid combining meat and dairy products at the same meal. Some Roman Catholics restrict meat consumption during Lent.

During the eighteenth and nineteenth centuries, people believed that eating fresh fruit caused serious illness, even death. During the cholera epidemic of 1848, the *Chicago Daily Journal* spread a fear of orchard-grown produce. Still another report claimed that a man who simply passed a fruit stand filled with spoiled peaches suffered a severe attack of the "gripes." Panic ensued, and people refused to eat fruit even after it was proven that the link between peaches and cholera wasn't the fruit itself, but the fruit-sellers' habit of washing their produce in polluted streams. This fear of fruit continued for many years.

In years gone by, a major fear of meat (apart from any underlying vegetarian or religious considerations) centered on its supposed association with "sexual excess." Other food superstitions were and are found around the globe. Pregnant women in the South Pacific islands, for example, weren't allowed to eat a certain type of shellfish because of fear that they would give birth to children with scales on their heads. Coffee was shunned because of a rumor that it was colored by horse blood. Even today, many rural Latin American women (and even some urban ones) have superstitions about diet during pregnancy, called "creencias." They believe that eating eggs during their pregnancy will kill their fetus because *they* are robbing a chicken of *its* life.

As late as 1940, dentist Melvin Page wrote in his book *Degeneration-Regeneration* that people shouldn't drink milk because it was "unnatural." He described milk as the underlying cause of colds, sinus infections, colitis, and cancer. In support of his theory he pointed to the dairy state of Wisconsin, which had a high rate of cancer deaths.

The "flip side" of the bad-food concept is the good-food panacea. History books identify a wide variety of foods that were believed to offer preventive and/or curative powers:

• Pliny recommended cucumbers for "hot stomachs and hot livers."

• Egyptians fed sick children skinned mice.

• Marcus Porcius Cato the Elder is reported to have believed so strongly in the magical powers of cabbage that he continued to eat it even after his "cabbage diet" failed to save the lives of his wife and son.

• In 1689 a prominent Italian physician promoted walnut

juice as a source of long life and health.

• In 1715 an English surgeon claimed that sugar alone could provide the basis for good nutrition, good disposition, and a cure for all wounds. (It's interesting to note that research has shown that applying sugar to some types of open wounds does promote healing.)

• Another eighteenth-century doctor recommended vinegar as a cure for yellow fever.

• A large group of would-be therapists based their advice on a belief that the outward characteristics of all plants and animals reflect the disease they are most useful in curing. Therefore, the lungs of the long-winded fox were recommended for asthma, the juice of a red beet for anemia, and the root of the mandrake (which is thought to resemble the two legs of a man) for male impotence. (There could be something to the mandrake root theory since its narcotic effect might decrease a lover's nervousness.) Primitive notions about herbs remain abundant in herbal guidebooks sold by "health food" stores today.

• Garlic has long been considered a superfood. In ancient Greece, Dioscorides claimed that garlic was excellent for cleaning out arteries and opening obstructions. However, he did warn that, if used in excess, it would stir up lust and provoke lechery. The Egyptians fed manual laborers large doses of garlic to keep them healthy and strong while they were building the pyramids. And during the 1940s, Adolphus Hohensee urged his audiences to put their faith in garlic for curing low blood pressure, inhibiting germs, cleansing blood, and cleaning out their intestines.

• Garlic wasn't the only popular "natural" laxative. Doses of sarsaparilla, molasses, and sulfur (which "cheered while it cured"), as well as good old-fashioned sea water, were even recommended in April or May as part of "spring cleaning."

Food Combinations

In addition to promoting the bad-food/good-food concept, self-proclaimed health experts have given advice on how to eat. In the 1920s, for example, some "experts" warned against eating carbohydrate and protein at the same meal. Others cautioned against combining acid and alkaline foods in the same meal for fear that these substances would interfere with each other's nutritional values. (The self-proclaimed experts forgot to mention that all foods become acidic when they are mixed with the stomach's hydrochloric acid.)

Twentieth-century health enthusiast Horace Fletcher (1849–1919) warned that "nature will castigate those who don't masticate." He recommended chewing foods at least thirty-two times, an action he assured would ensure absorption of all nutrients. Even liquids, he advocated, should be rolled around in the mouth a few times before being swallowed.

Fasting for Health

Fasting was often recommended to promote good health. Ancient Egyptians believed that diseases such as smallpox and measles were merely outward signs of food-related "corruption escaping the body." They would fast for a full three days each month to rid themselves of these poisons.

During the twentieth century, many popular books have recommended periods of fasting as a key to health. Hereward

Carrington's 1908 book *Vitality, Fasting and Nutrition* recommended regular fasting for good health. Upton Sinclair (1878–1968) followed up on Carrington's theory in 1911 with his own book *The Fasting Cure,* which recommends long periods of starvation as a means of combating tuberculosis, syphilis, asthma, liver trouble, and cancer. In a subsequent book, *The Book of Life,* Sinclair wrote: "I have known of two or three cases of people dying while they were fasting, but I feel quite certain that the fast did not cause their death, they would have died anyhow." Even today, "Natural Hygienists" advocate periodic fasting to help the body "purify and repair itself."

Graham Crackers, Corn Flakes, and the Return to the Garden of Eden

Many well-known individuals have espoused natural eating. Jean-Jacques Rousseau (1712–1778) commented that civilization made people evil and life "in the state of nature" was far superior to sophisticated lifestyles. Professor Carl von Linné, a Swedish contemporary of Rousseau, emphasized the nutritional aspects of "natural" living. He recommended that humans eat like their nearest animal-kingdom cousin, the ape, and concentrate on raw vegetables, berries and other fruits, milk, and roots.

Throughout the past two centuries, there has been no shortage of nutrition buffs to follow up on these early thoughts.

Sylvester Graham

Dr. Sylvester Graham (1794–1851) mixed religion with a zeal for the natural, "uncomplicated" life. A member of the Pennsylvania Temperance Society, he stated:

The simpler, plainer and more natural the food of Man is . . . the more healthy, vigorous and long lived will be the body, the more perfect will be all the senses, the more active and powerful may the intellectual and moral facilities be rendered by suitable cultivation.

Graham felt that a truly healthy diet included only what was available in the Garden of Eden: "fruits, nuts, farinaceous seeds and roots," occasionally supplemented by a bit of honey and milk. This eating style didn't allow any artificial preparation, except cracking the shells of nuts.

Graham's list of forbidden foods included salt and other condiments (since they, like sexual excess, caused insanity), cooked vegetables (which were against God's laws), tea (which caused delirium tremens), chicken pies (which were a source of cholera), and liquor (for obvious reasons!). But his most forceful and popular efforts were focused on avoidance of obviously "unnatural" substances (like meat and white flour products) and of bad eating habits (such as drinking water during a meal).

Graham's distaste for products made from white flour laid the groundwork for his entry into the business world. He began to market his own whole-wheat Graham flour, Graham bread, and the still-famous Graham cracker, all of which were highly praised in the *Graham Journal of Health and Longevity*. For best results, Graham recommended, his products should be eaten throughout the day, but never accompanied by water.

But Graham soon became his own worst enemy. He tended to be overly enthusiastic, to weaken his arguments by overstating them, and then began to support his arguments with examples too delicate for mixed company. When he lost his following, he shifted from the health food industry to writing poetry. He died at age fifty-seven, after "stimulants, a tepid bath, and a dose of congress waters."

John Harvey and William Kellogg

At least one avid follower lived out Graham's recommendations. John Harvey Kellogg (1852–1943) survived medical school on a diet of apples and Graham crackers. Around the turn of the century, Dr. Kellogg and his Seventh-day Adventist colleagues opened a religious colony and health sanitarium at Battle Creek, Michigan. Dr. Kellogg and his brother Will have been described as the first men to make a million dollars from food faddism.

The Kelloggs taught that it was God's law that man eat only plants and fruit. Dr. Kellogg served inpatients two "health foods." Granula (an early version of present-day granola) was made from leftover oven-dried bread that was subsequently ground. Zwieback was made from raised, sliced, and then overbaked bread. When a patient in the sanitarium broke his tooth on this diet (and demanded a very expensive replacement), the Kellogg brothers began searching for a more acceptable health food. "Wheat flakes" soon made their debut.

By 1899 Will Kellogg had built up a large corporation. The cereal-based health food industry was well established, and competitors began to sprout.

Charles W. Post

One of these competitors, Charles W. Post (1854–1914), was a former patient of the Kellogg sanitarium. He invented another type of ready-to-eat "health cereal" by baking wheat and barley loaves, drying them, and grinding them into small bits that resembled gravel. For some unexplained reason, Post called his creation "grape nuts" (although it contained neither grapes nor nuts) and marketed it as a cure for appendicitis, loose teeth, consumption, and malaria. A copy of his booklet "The Road to

Wellville" was included in every package of his product.

One of the largest segments of our modern food industry has grown from these first cereal "health foods." Although its origins involved faddism, the current breakfast-food industry, which includes the Kellogg Company, the Post Division of General Foods, General Mills, and several other companies, provides many nutritious food products, conducts excellent research, and sponsors outstanding public service activities.

Graham, Kellogg, and Post were tamer than many of the faddists who followed them.

Adolphus Hohensee

Adolphus Hohensee (1901–1967) began his "nutrition" career as a soda jerk. He then ventured into real estate and was successful until he strayed off the path to pass bad checks and dabble in mail fraud. Still seeking greener pastures the easy way, Hohensee obtained an Honorary Doctor of Medicine degree from the unaccredited Kansas City University School of Physicians and Surgeons. He received this degree in 1943, just a year before the institution was closed.

"Dr." Hohensee's health food business tactics were not original. He used scare tactics designed to cast doubt on the safety of regularly available food, followed by a spectacular presentation of his own products which, of course, were guaranteed to meet every need. A real showman, he often began by telling his audience that 90 percent of them had worms. Next, he vividly described the worms—two to twenty feet long, with their head in the victim's stomach and their body extending into the victim's intestines. Fortunately, listeners were assured, the Hohensee special cleansing diet could make them worm-free.

Then Hohensee would announce that due to a poor diet Americans suffered from poor health and were unable to perform sexually—a claim that he defined in detail. Those who didn't believe the worm scare perked up their ears with this presentation!

The average American diet, he continued in great detail, stagnated the blood, corroded the blood vessels, eroded the kidneys, and clogged the intestines. Food additives were the worst culprits, causing a type of slow poisoning process that inevitably followed the eating of "dead" processed foods. Hohensee portrayed himself as a noble individual being persecuted by such powerful enemies as "the American Murder Association," the Food and Drug Administration, the Better Business Bureau, and manufacturers of foods and drugs.

Hohensee recommended a three-step approach to ensure long life: (1) consume Hohensee-endorsed wonder products daily (which were available in the health food store next to the lecture hall), (2) avoid certain disease-causing foods (liquor, white bread, and particularly fried foods, and (3) use garlic suppositories regularly.

The FDA was long on Hohensee's trail, trying to knock him out of the health fraud business. After several attempts, the FDA and other regulatory agencies successfully fined Hohensee for misrepresenting his products. Like Graham, however, Hohensee was his own worst enemy. He was caught by the press consuming a gigantic meal of foods he himself had forbidden. Subsequent newspaper headlines read "What's Up, Doc?" and "'Nature Doc' Dines Out and Knocks a Decade off His 180-Year Life Span."

William Howard Hay

William Howard Hay, M.D., attributed most health problems to three dietary shortcomings, which he detailed in his 1933 book

Health Via Food. Americans, he said, eat too much protein, consume "adulterated" food like white bread, and retain food in the bowels for more than twenty-four hours after eating. He recommended changing the diet to reduce its protein content, eating "natural" foods, fasting, and frequent use of laxatives. He operated a sanitarium where the fare included Parcel Post Asparagus, Easter Bunny Salad, Fountain of Youth Salad, Hay's Happy Highball, and Pale Moon Cocktail (the latter two without alcohol).

Gayelord Hauser

Gayelord Hauser (1895–1984) believed that the "miracle of life" lay in the naturopathic approach. He gave many lectures and popularized his ideas in his book *Look Younger, Live Longer,* which made the nonfiction bestseller list in 1950 and led the list in 1951. With actress Greta Garbo as one of his major followers, Hauser recommended five wonder foods: skim milk, brewer's yeast, wheat germ, yogurt, and blackstrap molasses. Many people believed his claims that a diet of these foods would add years to their life. Following his death at age eighty-nine from complications of pneumonia, the *Los Angeles Times* reported that his fourteen books had sold nearly fifty million copies.

Lelord Kordel

Lelord Kordel (1904–) has written twenty books on "nutrition," including *Eat and Grow Younger* and *Eat Your Way to Happiness.* Early in his career he became president of Vital Foods, a "health food" company. He began producing and marketing dietary supplements, but was soon caught and fined for misbranding them. He claimed, for example, that one of his products could restore youth and "produce erect posture, sharp eyes, velvety skin, limbs of splendid proportions, deep chests, firm bodies, gracefully curved hips, flat abdomens (and) pleasing laughter." Other products were falsely claimed to treat heart disease, liver problems, tuberculosis, bone infections, and impotence. In 1963, while he still was president of Vital Foods, products shipped by the company were found to be misbranded because they were accompanied by Kordel publications that falsely claimed these nutritional products could treat practically all diseases. After the appeals process ended in 1971, Kordel was fined $10,000 and spent a year in prison.

Carlton Fredericks

Although Carlton Fredericks had no formal training in either nutrition or medicine, he found his niche in 1937 writing advertising for the U.S. Vitamin Corporation and giving talks as a "nutrition educator." He soon overstepped his bounds, however, and in 1945 paid a fine after pleading guilty to practicing medicine without a license. Ten years later he received his Ph.D. degree—still without ever having taken a nutrition course.

Fredericks is best known for his recommendations of dangerously high levels of vitamin A and his crusade against sugar. He consistently made false and misleading statements in his books and on talk shows, where he was introduced as a "leading nutrition consultant." Despite the scorn he endured by federal regulatory agencies, his personal charm and persuasive manner gave him undeserved credibility. He died from a heart attack in 1987 at the age of seventy-six. He had been a heavy smoker for most of his life.

D. C. Jarvis

D. C. Jarvis, M.D. (1881–1966), a general practitioner, made his contribution to the growing library of food faddism in 1958 with *Folk Medicine: A Vermont Doctor's Guide to Good Health,* a book that revived an eighteenth-century interest in vinegar. Dr. Jarvis believed that the principal threat to American health was an excess of "alkalinity." To increase acidity and create an environment that would prevent "the infestation of the body with pathogenic microorganisms," patients were advised to avoid meat, wheat and wheat-containing foods, citrus fruits, white sugar, and maple sugar—and dose themselves with two tablespoons of apple cider vinegar before each meal. Dr. Jarvis further advised a daily urine check to measure the progress in the battle against alkalinity. Needless to say, there is no scientific basis for these beliefs.

J. I. Rodale

Jerome Irving Rodale (1898–1971), the undisputed father of twentieth-century Healthfoodland, began his business career as a manufacturer of electrical wiring accessories. But he switched to promoting natural, "organic" living after reading what British agronomist Sir Albert Howard had to say about achieving a healthy lifestyle. Like Howard, Rodale began to preach that eating "God's way" was necessary to remain healthy and ensure a long life.

Rodale's doctrines came to include several points. First, only natural, organic matter should be used to fertilize the soil. Unlike prepared chemical fertilizer, organic material supposedly guaranteed that the soil would hold moisture and retain its "tillability." Furthermore, organic farming methods (as opposed to "artificial means") were said to provide more basic, balanced nutrients for plants.

Second, said Rodale, foods should be eaten directly—raw and without adding anything artificial. He justified this belief by stating that "no animal eats cooked food."

Third, certain foods should be avoided at all cost. He railed against wheat (because it made a person overaggressive and "daffy") and sugar (even worse than wheat and to be shunned by all organic eaters). And he said that fluoridated water should be avoided even if it meant buying bottled water.

Fourth, it was essential to supplement one's diet with rose hips, natural vitamins and minerals, and other such health-enhancers each day. Mr. Rodale and his wife reportedly took seventy food supplement tablets each day.

Rodale's nutritional advice was promoted both through his books (including *Organic Front, Happy People Rarely Get Cancer,* and *Sugar and the Criminal Mind*) and in magazines and newsletters that regularly rolled off the Rodale Press. Although the American Medical Association regularly included Rodale publications in its quackery exhibits, Rodale's publishing venture maintained a faithful following. The best-known Rodale publication, *Prevention* magazine was launched in 1950 and now boasts a circulation in excess of three million, while its number-two magazine, *Organic Gardening,* has more than one million subscribers.

J. I. Rodale insisted that his healthy lifestyle would enable him to live to one hundred years of age unless he was "run down by a sugar-crazed taxi driver," but he died at age seventy-two while taping an interview for the Dick Cavett Show. (A detailed biography written after Rodale's death says that for several months he had been having attacks of chest pain and rapid pulse.) J. I.'s son Robert inherited the Rodale empire and, among other things, served as editor-in-chief of *Prevention* for many years.

During the mid-1980s, *Prevention* began changing its editorial policy and even recruited some well-known enemies of health quackery as advisors. In the process, it advanced from an "unreliable" rating in the 1984 American Council on Science and Health's survey of nutrition reporting in magazines to ratings of "inconsistent" in 1986 and "fair" in 1988. *Prevention* editors now send the majority of articles out for professional review prior to publication, and its accuracy has improved further. It recommends eating a balanced diet and no longer attributes magical properties to foods or food supplements. It exhorts its readers to maintain a healthy lifestyle that includes regular exercise and excludes cigarette smoking. Be aware, however, that *Prevention* still carries misleading ads and that many books marketed by Rodale Press and its Prevention Book Club remain firmly entrenched in health faddism.

Adelle Davis

According to Adelle Davis (1904–1974), proper diet not only prevents and cures virtually any disease, but can have important effects on the quality of life of society as a whole. Unlike most of the faddists who preceded her, Ms. Davis received a "proper" nutrition education, acquiring a degree in nutrition and dietetics from the University of California at Berkeley and an M.S. degree in biochemistry from the University of Southern California Medical School. Unfortunately, she strayed from fact into fiction and became a major contributor to "panic in the pantry."

Adelle Davis advised her followers to avoid refined sugar, pasteurized or homogenized milk, white bread, food additives, "unfertile" eggs, and any food that might have come in contact with "chemical fertilizers." For Ms. Davis, "proper diet" meant focusing on whole grains, fresh milk, fruits, and vegetables. She disagreed with the prevailing medical opinion that saturated fats and cholesterol should be consumed in moderation, and she advocated eating at least two (fertile) eggs every day.

Ms. Davis wrote numerous articles and four popular books: *Let's Eat Right to Keep Fit, Let's Cook It Right, Let's Get Well,* and *Let's Have Healthy Children.* She also lectured and made television appearances, all in an effort to promote her ideas. "A woman," she gravely warned, "who wants to murder her husband can do it through the kitchen. There won't even be an inquest."

Adelle Davis impressed her listeners and readers by citing thousands of respectable-sounding references to back up her statements and advice. In *Let's Get Well,* for example, she listed 2,402 references to document thirty-four chapters. Although her work might appear to be very well researched, when Dr. Edward H. Rynearson, professor emeritus of medicine at the Mayo Clinic and Mayo Foundation, actually attempted to track down the "references" for some of her statements, he found that a significant number of her comments had no basis at all. In chapter 12 of *Let's Get Well,* for instance, he found that twenty-seven of the fifty-seven references contained no data to support her statements. Dr. George Mann of the Department of Biochemistry and Medicine at Vanderbilt University School of Medicine analyzed her most popular book, *Let's Eat Right to Keep Fit,* and found an average of one mistake per page.

Despite the unreliability of her advice, a 1972 Associated Press article said she "is to nutrition what Ralph Nader is to consumerism." Many physicians, however, expressed grave concerned about her misleading advice. For example, when she took a position against bottle-feeding and stated that crib deaths could be prevented by breast-feeding and dietary supplements of vitamin E, at least one physician responded by sending a letter of complaint to the Federal Communications Commission, asking for immediate action. Ms. Davis replied to this physician's inquiry by writing, "Thank you so much for correcting me. I am indeed sorry if words of mine have added to the suffering of parents whose infants have died." Her retraction, however, received very little public attention.

In *Let's Get Well,* Ms. Davis recommended that patients with nephrosis take potassium chloride, a suggestion that medical specialists labeled "extremely dangerous and even potentially lethal." Recommendations in *Let's Have Healthy Children* are known to have had tragic results. In 1976 the estate of Adelle Davis paid a $150,000 settlement to the family of a child whose growth was permanently stunted by large doses of vitamin A, as recommended in *Let's Have Healthy Children.* And in 1978 an infant had died from the administration of potassium chloride for colic as recommended in the same book. To settle lawsuits brought by the child's parents, Ms. Davis's estate paid $75,000, the publisher $25,000, and the potassium manufacturer $60,000. Unfortunately, little public notice was taken of these tragedies. The publisher stopped marketing the book but had it revised by a physician aligned with the health food industry. The newer version is filled with unfounded advice about supplements but appears far less dangerous than the original.

At age sixty-nine, Adelle Davis learned she had multiple myeloma, a cancer of the bone marrow. She was shocked that she could develop such a disease despite all of her attention to healthful living. In an interview in *Let's Live* magazine, she attributed her cancer to three things: (1) dietary indiscretions (consuming enriched bread, pasteurized milk, and "junk food") during the middle third of her life, (2) a very heavy work schedule, and (3) "too many x-rays," which had been taken during the previous year because her sponsors wanted to have her insured. Just before her death, she urged her followers not to lose heart, but to continue to seek long life and good health through "natural" products.

Lendon Smith

Pediatrician Lendon H. Smith, M.D., became a household name through his book *Feed Your Kids Right,* which claimed that hyperactivity in children, allergies, insomnia, alcoholism, and a variety of other conditions were the result of disturbances in the body's enzymes and could be helped by changes in diet. He recommended avoiding white sugar, white flour, pasteurized milk, and other "unnatural" foods and using supplements at levels that are proven to be dangerous. Dr. Smith wrote ten books and, largely due to his humorous style of delivery, was a frequent talk show guest.

In 1973 the Oregon Board of Medical Examiners ordered Smith to surrender his narcotics license and placed him on a ten-year probation after Smith prescribed narcotics to heroin addicts. They also ordered him to limit his practice to treating children. After this action was taken, he turned away from traditional medicine and adopted "nutritional therapy," working primarily with naturopaths, homeopaths, and chiropractors. The narcotics restriction was relaxed somewhat in 1974 but was reapplied in 1975. His probation lasted until 1981.

In January 1987 Smith permanently surrendered his medical license to avoid another conflict with the Oregon Board of Medical Examiners. He had been charged with violating two Oregon state laws—"obtaining any fee by fraud or misrepresentation" and "making a fraudulent claim" related to the billing of insurance companies for services by his associates. He still writes for some faddist publications but appears to have little public impact.

Paavo Airola

The biographical blurbs on the jackets of Paavo Airola's books describe him as holding Ph.D. and N.D. degrees but neglect to mention where his education took place. Eleven of his fourteen books are sold to health food stores by Health Plus Publishers, a division of Airola, Inc. The books stress the use of herbs, juices, natural foods, vitamins, minerals, and other supplements to treat more than sixty conditions and illnesses. Promotional material accompanying these books and directed to the store owners points out the substantial amount of money to be made by selling the items Airola recommends to readers interested in self-treatment.

Airola claimed that humans should live to the age of 120 unless they "kill themselves prematurely by violating the basic laws of health and life." Despite this, he died in 1983 at the age of sixty-four.

Harvey and Marilyn Diamond

Fit for Life (1985), by self-proclaimed nutritionists Harvey and Marilyn Diamond, has been described by consumer advocate and health-fraud specialist Stephen Barrett, M.D., as containing more silly ideas and misinformation than any other "nutrition" book he has ever seen. The book states that the Diamonds hold credentials in "nutrition science" and "nutrition counseling" from the American College of Health Science—an unaccredited correspondence school that was later ordered by a Texas court to stop calling itself a college or issuing "degrees."

The Diamonds' erroneous beliefs include: (1) eating foods in the wrong combinations causes them to rot so that they can't be assimilated, (2) some foods cleanse the body while others clog it, (3) the main cause of overweight is an accumulation of "toxic waste" from the incomplete digestion and assimilation of food, (4) eggs rot in the body, and (5) fruits and vegetables, because of their high water content, can be used to wash the body and cleanse it from toxins. In addition to their "bad science," the Diamonds recommend a diet that is low in calcium and can result in deficiencies in other essential nutrients.

Durk Pearson and Sandy Shaw

Pearson and Shaw's 1982 book *Life Extension: A Practical Scientific Approach* appealed to many people who wanted to extend their life; so many, in fact, that it became a bestseller. Authors Durk Pearson and Sandy Shaw differ from most food faddists in that they don't condemn additives and "unnatural" chemicals. In fact, their own published formula contains more than thirty food supplements and prescription drugs. Pearson and Shaw's statement that they don't actually recommend their program for "anyone but themselves" is probably the most responsible piece of information in this absurd book. Among other things, they recommend that you can determine your proper dose of a drug by slowly increasing the amount you take until you reach "an unacceptable level of the type of harmless and reversible side effects you can get with megadoses of these low toxicity nutrients." However, the authors fail to explain how to identify which side effects are both harmless and reversible. Dr. Stephen Barrett found little in the book that could be labeled "good science" and has estimated that the recommended program would cost thousands of dollars a year. This so-called life extension program appears to be neither practical nor scientific.

Further Shaping Public Attitude . . . United We Stand

Many food faddists and nutrition alarmists have found strength in numbers. One of the largest such groups is the National Health Federation (NHF), a health food industry group founded in 1955. NHF promotes a wide range of unproven and dubious health products and practices. More than a dozen of its present or former leaders have had many brushes with the law.

NHF founder Fred J. Hart, president of the Electronic Medical Foundation, was fined in 1962 for violating a 1954 court order barring his company from distributing bogus medical devices.

The most notorious of NHF's officers was probably Kurt W. Donsbach, a chiropractor who chaired its board of governors for more than ten years. In 1970, while operating a health food store, Donsbach pleaded guilty to practicing medicine without a license and agreed to stop his "nutritional consultations." Three years later, he sold the company that had manufactured many of the products he had recommended in his "consultations."

During the late 1970s, Donsbach began offering B.S., M.S., and Ph.D. "degrees" in nutrition through Donsbach University, an unaccredited school that operated mainly by mail. He also helped establish the International Institute of Natural Health Sciences, which, for several years, published booklets recommending "supplement products" for a large number of diseases and conditions. Today he administers a clinic in Mexico that offers unproven treatments for cancer and other serious diseases.

NHF is perhaps best known for its lobbying activities on behalf of the health food industry, including its ability to launch massive letter-writing campaigns to influence Congress.

"Nutrition Activists"

A 1970 book attacking the FDA, *The Chemical Feast,* was written by consumer-activist Ralph Nader and two colleagues. *The Chemical Feast* promoted the idea that health problems in the U.S. were the result of an unsafe food supply. One of Nader's colleagues was attorney James Turner, who, during 1978, was identified as NHF's "Washington representative."

In 1971, a trio of Naderites formed the Center for Science in the Public Interest (CSPI). CSPI's stated goal is the investigation and reporting of food and food chemical issues. Microbiologist Michael Jacobson edits CSPI's monthly newsletter. Unfortunately, some of CSPI's ideas sound all too familiar: "chemical farming methods create environmental havoc," "every few months, it seems, another common food additive is found to be harmful," and "most Americans get their information about food from ads by the big food corporations, which are ... more concerned with big profits than with good nutrition." CSPI typically oversimplifies and sensationalizes issues concerning the food supply, almost inevitably concluding that what we eat isn't safe—a stance that aids and abets both food faddism and the health food industry.

To be fair, we must also note that CSPI has taken some very positive and successful actions against misleading advertising of certain foods and dietary supplements.

The Bottom Line

Unfortunately, not much has changed since an early publication of this century, *Stover at Yale,* described a handy blueprint for promoting patent medicines and becoming a millionaire in ten years. It applies equally as well to fad nutrition products:

> First, find something all the fools love and enjoy, tell them it's wrong, hammer it into them, give them a substitute, and sit back, chuckle, and shovel away the ducats. Why, in the next 20 years, all the fools will be feeding on substitutes for everything they want . . . and blessing the name of the foolmaster who fooled them.

Marketing of health food, then, continues to provide substantial profits for those who succeed in taking advantage of the public's deep-seated fears about illness and their quest for good, if not superior, health. Groucho Marx once asked a health food promoter on his radio show what his product was good for. With unusual candor, the health food promoter replied, "It was good for about five and a half million last year."

And, as we'll read in the next chapter, promoting health food is still good for millions today.

3

The Garden of Eden: '70s and '80s Style

"It seems a shame," the Walrus said,
"To play them such a trick,
After we've brought them out so far,
And made them trot so quick!"
The Carpenter said nothing but
"The butter's spread too thick!"

—Lewis Carroll
Through the Looking Glass

There's Money in Honey!

America's preoccupation with organic and additive-free food is entering its third decade. Sylvester Graham would have been pleased—and probably a bit envious—at the health food movement's current popularity.

In the 1830s, when Graham began marketing his version of food faddism, he was pretty much alone. Most of his customers were people who attended his lectures, subscribed to his journal, or responded to local newspaper ads. The parade of food faddists who lectured their way through the next century also had limited followings. The early "health food" movement

41

hooked the emotions of a relatively small proportion of American eaters.

During the past twenty years, however, health foods and supplements have become big business. Natural products now cover the alphabet from asparagus to zwieback—with cosmetics, cookware, and even liquor and cigarettes falling somewhere in between. The trade magazine *Health Foods Business*, which conducts an annual survey, estimates that in 1991 there were 7,300 health food stores, with total sales of $3.88 billion. Vitamins and other supplements accounted for $1.46 billion of this figure. But many of the same wonder-products are hawked beyond the confines of health food stores. You can pick them up at the corner drugstore and your favorite supermarket; you can even make selections from the comfort of your easy chair, a service offered by person-to-person salespeople. Retail sales of supplements through other outlets are probably at least $2 billion a year.

Today's Bill of Fare

The philosophy of natural organic eating is based on four main assumptions, which are the cornerstones of Healthfoodland:

1. Organically grown food is more nutritious and is safer.
2. Some foods have magical properties.
3. "Natural" is always better than "artificial."
4. Vitamins and other food supplements can work wonders, and you aren't likely to get too much of a good thing.

These ideas have no basis in science and fact. We'll examine the first two in this chapter and the others in chapters 4 and 5.

Products From A to Z

Today, health food stores sell more than just vitamins and minerals. Their many products include: bottled water; herbs and herbal teas; "natural" bodycare items; "natural" grains and cereals; "natural" nuts, seeds, and beans; "organic" fruits and vegetables; "natural" snacks and confections; additive-free and hormone-free meat products; fish raised in "unpolluted" water; amino acids; mixtures to slim you down, "bulk" you up, calm you down, pep you up, increase your fiber, and decrease your gas problem (caused by increasing your fiber?); homeopathic "remedies"; exercise equipment; and books about the products sold in the stores.

Most stores no longer provide the option of picking up raw milk as you wander up and down the aisles. About half the states now ban the sale of unpasteurized milk, and the FDA has prohibited its transport for sale across state lines. If you're still willing to take the serious health risks associated with drinking raw milk (discussed later in this book), you have a choice: either find a dairy farmer willing to take the chance of selling it or follow the advice of some natural food enthusiasts and get milk from your own cow—a step guaranteed to make you unpopular in most neighborhoods. Of course, if you don't mind your "milk" in solid form and from a tiger, you can still purchase products bearing the familiar Tiger's Milk label. This old health food standby (which is neither milk nor from a tiger) is now primarily sold as nutrition bars.

The label of a *Tiger's Milk Nutrition Bar* lists the following ingredients: corn syrup, brown sugar, peanut butter, nonfat dry milk, partially hydrogenated vegetable oil (soybean, cottonseed), soy bean isolate, soy flour, sodium caseinate, carob powder, water, tricalcium phosphate, lecithin, natural vanilla, ascorbic acid, ferrous fumarate, niacin, calcium, pantothenate, copper gluconate, vitamin A palmitate, pyridoxine hydrochloride, thiamine, monocitrate, riboflavin, vitamin D from fish liver oils, biotin, and cyanocobalamin. Health food enthusiasts who take the time to read the label (should you have to do that in a health food store?) will no doubt be surprised at all of the strange-sounding chemicals in their "health" food!

Perhaps the most fascinating area of the health food store is the supplement section. Contradictory as it seems, few naturalists rely on food alone—even if it is 100 percent organic and additive-free. They need vitamins, minerals, protein supplements, desiccated liver, wheat germ oil, and a whole collection of other supposedly life-giving (and expensive) products.

Another part of the "natural" lifestyle is a regular cleaning out. Obligingly, health food stores feature several dozen different types of laxatives, ranging from sea water to products that are often made of papain, whey, and alfalfa (at times advertised as a means of "cultivating your inner organic garden"). The more extreme health enthusiast may also "clean house" with high colonic enemas. Harvey and Marilyn Diamond, authors of *Fit for Life*, propose an even easier way that seems *truly* natural. All you have to do is eat fruits and vegetables, which, having a high water content, "wash out" the body from the inside!

Truth is Stranger than Fiction: "Natural Vices"

Strange as it may seem, cigarette manufacturers have climbed aboard the back-to-nature bandwagon, offering more "natural" cigarettes. Because cigarette smoking has been unequivocally identified as the one single most preventable cause of premature death in the United States, it's difficult to see how it can be linked with health in any way. Interestingly, the tobacco industry doesn't have to identify the additives in its products (unless they advise you to eat their cigarettes, thereby bringing them under FDA jurisdiction!).

Liquor, too, has managed to get into the act. Several years ago Dr. Frederic Damrau and Professor Arthur H. Goldberg at Columbia University's School of Pharmaceutical Sciences confirmed that the "additives" or congeners (esters and other impurities in some alcoholic beverages that give liquor its flavor) and not the alcohol itself cause a hangover. This led to an immediate rush on "natural" cocktails made, of course, with vodka—alcohol reduced to its natural (and tasteless) state by filtering it through charcoal.

Tests conducted with volunteers confirmed that individuals drinking vodka suffered significantly fewer hangover symptoms—irritation of the stomach and lower gastrointestinal tract, headache, dizziness, and fatigue—than subjects drinking non-charcoal-filtered alcohol. On the other hand, more than half the test subjects who received as little as one ounce of "zero proof" whiskey—made by removing the alcohol and leaving only water and congeners—had hangover symptoms. A number of medical researchers have confirmed this observation—a fact apparently known to the Russians years ago. Because most people in this country like the taste, bouquet, and color of whiskey, vodka has yet to dominate the liquor market.

Natural Looking

If you treat your inside to natural goodness, why not your outside, too? This reasoning is the basis of the natural cosmetic industry, which manufactures a rather elaborate selection of "natural" health-care products. Some of them sound almost good enough to eat! You can choose from creamy milk bath; honey shampoo; wheat germ, yeast, or avocado beauty masks; vitamin hair tonics; cucumber, coconut oil, tomato, or "milk and honey" soap; and, for dessert, a choice of strawberry, peach, or apple cleanser for your skin.

"Look younger." (An approach guaranteed to appeal to a large segment of the population.) "Go natural." There's very little difference between today's advertising campaigns and yesterday's invitations to wash your hair with *Herbal Essence* shampoo and "launch on a totally new experience" with Elizabeth Arden's multiple-action cleansing cream ("suddenly your face feels invigorated with a look of natural health"). Why pollute your face with artificial goo when you can pay a premium price for "natural" goo?

Don't Drink the Water Unless It's Natural

What could be more natural than the water you drink? Not so, say those individuals making a good living from the growing business of distributing home water filters and purifiers. Their brochures aren't really educational—they're just good old-fashioned "hard sell" based on scaring consumers into parting with more of their hard-earned money. Some filters are not very effective or become clogged too soon, rendering them ineffective. Some can even become breeding grounds for bacteria.

Bottled water has become a desirable commodity in American grocery stores. Many brands provide a legitimate alternative for people who dislike the taste of their community water supply (or water from their own well). However, it is inappropriate for bottlers to make health claims for their products or to frighten people away from perfectly good tap water.

What Do "Organic," "Natural," Etc., Really Mean?

Several elements of the health food movement make it an ideal setting for fraud. First, there are no meaningful definitions for "organic," "natural," and similar terms used throughout Healthfoodland. Second, there isn't any practical way to identify foods that have been grown "organically." Third, and probably most important, health-oriented people who dig deep into their pockets to pay for these products are both loyal and unsuspecting.

"Organic foods" (also called "organically grown foods") are said by their proponents to be foods grown without the use of pesticides or "chemical" fertilizers. Scientists (and ordinary dictionaries) use the word "organic" to refer to compounds that contain carbon bonded to other atoms in certain ways—which would apply to all foods that come from living organisms. All foods composed of carbohydrate, protein, and/or fat are organic by their very nature. So, calling a particular type of food "organic" (suggesting, of course, that others are not) is like labeling water from a particular source "wet." Nonetheless, "organic" proponents have succeeded in getting laws passed to set "definitions" and "standards" in about half the states. At one point even the FDA drafted a definition, which prompted an FDA attorney to remark that most of the definitions, "including ours, are sheer nonsense."

The term "natural food" is usually intended to mean a product produced and marketed with little if any processing and that is free of preservatives, antibiotics, emulsifiers, additives, or other added ingredients. Scientists have pointed out that this definition is ambiguous because all of our foods are natural or manufactured from natural foods. Individual nutrients, such as vitamins or additives, either may be naturally occurring or manufactured synthetically.

"Health foods" are said to be special foods that improve a person's health. This general term includes foods labeled "natural," "dietetic," "organic," or "vegetarian." However, all foods, when eaten in moderation, can contribute to health. No matter where you buy them, any foods eaten in excess can accurately be called "unhealth" foods.

During the mid-1970s the Federal Trade Commission (FTC) briefly considered banning commercial use of the terms "organic" or "organically grown," "natural," and "health" food. But an outcry from proponents caused the agency to abandon this idea and to consider setting standards for the terms "organic" and "natural." This concept was opposed by the scientific community because it would have been interpreted by the public as an FTC stamp of approval of the food myths associated with these products.

There's also the practical problem of enforcement. It would be very difficult to allocate funds for testing foods sold in health food establishments to see whether they comply with the terms used to describe them. Years ago New York Attorney General Louis J. Lefkowitz looked into complaints on this very issue. Investigators from the Bureau of Consumer Frauds and Protection shopped anonymously in about twenty-five health food stores in New York City. First they asked merchants to describe the benefits of their products over more traditional foods. The investigators were told that the health foods were pesticide-free, more nutritious, and generally healthier in the long run. Dr. Elmer George, who was director of the New York State Food Laboratory, then tested more than fifty "natural," "pesticide-free" items. He found that 30 percent of them contained pesticide residue, as compared to 20 percent of the regular foods.

Science and reason finally were defeated, however, when Congress passed the U.S. Organic Foods Production Act of 1990 (Title 21 of the 1990 Farm Bill). This legislation calls for:

the U.S. Secretary of Agriculture to set certification standards for organic foods; establishment of a 15-member National Organic Standards Board to suggest guidelines; a National List of substances permitted or prohibited for organic use; certification of organic farmers, processors, manufacturers, and wholesalers; labeling and record-keeping requirements; collection of fees from producers, certifiers, and handlers of organic foods; and civil penalties for violations of the Act of up to $10,000. In one senseless action, Congress legitimized the organic foods industry and countered the effect of years of painstaking public education about the uselessness of purchasing so-called organic foods.

The new law won't alter the fact that even farmers trying their best to use "organic" methods can end up with pesticides in their crops. It's almost impossible to avoid chemical residues since they can be deposited by wind and water. Also, there's no way of testing a food product to determine what kind of fertilizer was actually used. So you're left with a situation where certain specialty foods are being sold at a significantly higher price without any way to detect if they are "frauds."

In fact, many sellers have ripped off their own loyal health food enthusiasts by representing foods obtained from conventional sources as "organic." One case in point might be called the "counterfeit carrot caper." In 1988 the *San Francisco Chronicle* reported that carrots packaged by Pacific Organics were actually everyday supermarket carrots that were being transferred to clear cellophane and marketed as "organically grown."

There's also the question of "natural" and "organic" fertilizer used to produce "natural" and "organic" food. There are some differences between "natural" fertilizer (usually animal manure or green compost) and commercially prepared products—but not what you might think. Advocates of organic methods may state that the fertilizers used to grow their foods are, by nature, rich in the minerals that help plants reach full growth, while the commercial varieties are sadly lacking and contaminated with artificial ingredients.

The facts just don't agree! All fertilizers, whether commercially processed or from living organisms, must be broken down to their inorganic components, such as phosphorus, potassium, and nitrogen, before plants can absorb them. Actually, the "natural" variety takes a bit longer to do the job since it has to be chemically changed by bacteria in the soil before plants can use it. Once the substances in fertilizer have reached this stage, plants aren't able to identify their original source.

So the source of a fertilizer—"natural" or "artificial"—has no bearing on the quality of the plants it nourishes. Chemicals are chemicals no matter how they're supplied. However, this doesn't mean that these fertilizers are exactly alike. Natural fertilizer may lack some types of nutrients necessary for ideal farming conditions. Processed fertilizers, on the other hand, are of consistent quality and can be specially formulated to correct for any deficiency of a particular soil.

A "plus" for organic fertilizer is that it does improve the workability of the soil. However, it may also provide a very unwelcome "extra" missing in chemical fertilizers. Harmful organisms present in human or animal feces can find their way into the crops on which manure is applied, contributing opportunities for some real health problems that are easily avoided with conventional farming and food processing methods. Dr. Jean Mayer, a long-time professor of nutrition at Harvard, now president of Tufts University, pointed out:

> Biologically speaking, they [organic foods] tend to become the most contaminated of all. Organic fertilizers of animal or human origin are obviously the most likely to contain gastrointestinal parasites.

The sobering truth of this statement was driven home by reports from South Korea and Holland at a time when human sewage was used to fertilize crops. During this period, significant portions of the populations in both countries suffered from roundworm, hookworm, and other parasites. These diseases were the result of the improper use of organic fertilizer and an incomplete chemical breakdown of human and animal wastes. With commercially processed fertilizer, there's no such risk.

The claim that "organic foods" are nutritionally superior is also unfounded. An apple is an apple. Its vitamin content can't be altered by changing the way it's grown. The amount of vitamin C in an apple, for example, can't be increased to the level found in an orange by adding any amount of commercial fertilizer or other chemical stimulant. A food's vitamin content is largely determined by genetics and can be changed only by developing a new hybrid or strain. (The mineral content of foods is affected by the mineral content of the soil in which they are grown. But since plants are not the major source of minerals in our diet, this has no practical significance.)

Pesticide—Friend or Foe?

Natural food enthusiasts are adamantly opposed to pesticides. These people, however, overlook the very basic fact of life that mankind competes with the insect kingdom for food. And on many occasions, based on pure numbers alone, the insects have been known to win. It's been estimated that one pair of insects could produce 191 quadrillion hungry descendants in a single summer season if all of its offspring lived and reproduced normally. The use of pesticides makes farming efficient and helps keep consumer prices down.

The idea that poisons in pesticide sprays will somehow be

transferred to human food has been blown far out of proportion. Pesticide use is regulated by government codes specifying the amount of residue that may be present in the final products. These amounts are so small that they would have to be multiplied a hundredfold or more to reach a level that might possibly be harmful to human beings.

Under its regulatory monitoring program, the FDA collects samples from individual lots of both domestically grown and imported food and analyzes them for pesticide residues. The FDA also does a Total Diet Study (also called the Market Basket Study) to estimate the dietary intakes of pesticide residues for eight age-sex groups from infants to senior citizens.

Nearly twenty thousand food samples were tested by the FDA in 1990. Ninety-nine percent of the domestic samples contained no illegal residues, i.e., fewer than 1 percent of the samples had residues exceeding tolerances set by the Environmental Protection Agency (EPA). Sixty percent had no residues at all. In the imported samples, less than one percent had over-tolerance residues, 4 percent had residues for which there was no tolerance set, and 64 percent had no detectable residues. The 1990 Total Diet Study once again indicated that any residues found were well below the acceptable daily intakes established by the United Nations' Food and Agriculture Organization and World Health Organization.

As we'll see later, if people insist on worrying about food safety, they would do well to concentrate on the risk from carcinogens naturally occurring in food rather than on pesticide residues!

So Where's the Magic?

Health food enthusiasts are convinced that select "health" foods have magical properties. Although claims for "miracle foods" have no scientific basis, the term "health food" suggests otherwise.

This is nothing new. Whether it's Cato the Elder, who believed in cabbage, or later health faddists who concentrated on honey and wheat germ, the message is the same. In 1958 Dr. D. C. Jarvis, the Vermont country doctor, recommended apple cider and honey "to start the fat-burning process." If this sounds familiar, it is because the notion is still with us today. Instead of apple cider, more modern-day faddists may recommend grapefruit. Of course, for people who don't want to risk being squirted in the eye by a real, natural grapefruit, there are grapefruit tablets to provide the same imaginary benefits. No matter what the next "miracle fat-burning" food turns out to be, the one sure bet is that this money-making gimmick will always be around in one form or another.

Honey continues to hold its position as a leading miracle food. As one enthusiastic health food store owner said, "I recommend it [honey] for ulcers, cancers, and mostly for healthy people as a preventive of both." Others proclaim it as a "sure cure" for sore throats, coughs, and colds.

One honey-related product that caught public attention several years ago and that remains a big seller today is "royal jelly." This "glandular secretion made by worker bees for the queen bee" has been described in advertising as a "tonic for the nervous system," "a cure for nutritional problems of aging," and as a source of nutrients "thought to be necessary for energy, mental alertness, and a general feeling of well being." Supposedly, a group meeting in Rumania in 1983 reported that royal jelly was effective for tiredness and overwork, weakness, insomnia, anxiety, lack of appetite, bronchial asthma, liver diseases (hepatitis), pancreatitis, general exhaustion, arthritis, gout, atherosclerosis, kidney diseases, stomach ulcers, ovarian insufficiency, reversing the aging process, stimulating and regenerating the nervous system, speeding up the healing of broken bones, and skin disorders. (About the only condition not mentioned was hoof-and-mouth disease.)

Wheat germ also has received its share of undocumented credits. One company claimed that wheat kernels are effective in treating neuritis, arthritis, and constipation. Since there wasn't a grain of truth in this statement, the FDA quickly moved against that group. (Needless to say, federal agencies have their hands full dealing with false advertising and labeling of "health" foods and "food supplements" for the full gamut of diseases. Unfortunately, the FDA doesn't have nearly enough personnel to deal with these problems.)

Garlic tablets and a variety of other garlic-based products, including croutons, crackers, and garlic oil (for healthier arteries), are highly recommended by employees in health food stores. In spite of a paucity of scientific evidence, garlic continues to be recommended for treating heart disease, stroke, cancer, and bacterial infection. Trying some of these products "just in case they might do some good," however, may pose a significant health hazard. In mid-1989 the FDA told manufacturers to stop producing chopped garlic-in-oil mixes that require refrigeration. When left at room temperature, these products could grow *Clostridium botulinum,* the bacterium leading to botulism, a possibly fatal type of food poisoning. The FDA told manufacturers that to be safe they must add substances such as phosphoric or citric acid (chemicals!) that would inhibit bacterial growth.

Industrial Giants Enter the Picture

In the beginning, so-called natural products were primarily found in small, out-of-the-way outlets that carried brands familiar only to dedicated eaters of health food. This certainly isn't the case today. The health food business has become so big and so popular that it has drawn in some big players. Many food companies have found it easier and more profitable to jump on the back-to-nature bandwagon, cashing in on myths about natural foods, than to fight such food faddism with facts.

The natural cereals market is a stark example of how the food giants have been drawn in. Some major food companies have given that old stand-by, granola, some very fancy names—and prices—in response to consumer demands for natural cereal. Early entrants into the field included *Quaker 100% Natural Cereal* from Quaker Oats, *Heartland* from Pet, Inc., *Nature Valley* from General Mills, and *Country Morning* from Kellogg. When *Quaker 100% Natural Cereal* had been on the market for just a few weeks, a company representative said "It was obvious we were riding a tiger." The company was forced to cut back on advertising because it couldn't keep up with the demand.

A lot of "granola" cereals have been crunched since the beginning of the natural cereal boom. However, once consumers caught on to the fact that what most characterized granola cereals was added fat and sugar—giving more calories for less cereal—manufacturers often deleted the word granola from the name. To be sure of what you're buying, read the nutrition portion of the label.

Old standbys like *Kellogg's Corn Flakes* and *Post Bran Flakes* provide a reasonable amount of cereal per one-ounce, 130-calorie serving: one cup of corn flakes and 2/3 cup of bran flakes. Both of these cereals contain some added sugar but no fat. Compare with *Quaker 100% Natural Oats and Honey Cereal,* which also provides 130 calories per ounce. One ounce of this "natural" cereal is only 1/4 cup (a *very* small bowl) and contains six grams (equal to 54 calories) of fat. Reading the nutrition information on the label is the only way to identify the cereals that provide a lot of fat and calories in a relatively small serving. And one thing Americans don't need more of is calories!

Bad Attitudes About Good Additives

Food manufacturers often use "natural" on the label of products to which they have stopped adding compounds—additives— intended to protect safety and prolong freshness. This trend toward "naturalness" in our food supply could lead to more serious problems than extra poundage.

There are good reasons why preservatives and other types of additives are used in food. Take bread, for example. For many years bread has contained the preservative calcium propionate to prevent it from molding. Since calcium propionate does not occur naturally in bread's ingredients, it must be labeled an additive (and therefore be suspect). Of course, most people already consume some calcium propionate, since it is a "natural" product of the fermentation process in making Swiss cheese. So what will you get in bread labeled "no artificial preservatives"? The label of *Flowers Nature's Own Soft Natural Grains Bread* with "no artificial preservatives, colors, or flavors" says: "dough conditioners—contains one or more of the following (sodium stearoyl-2-lactylate, calcium stearoyl-2-lactylate, mono- and diglycerides, ethoxylated mono- and diglycerides, potassium bromate, monocalcium phosphate, ammonium sulfate, ferrous sulfate. . ."

There is no reason to be nervous about the unfamiliar chemical names listed above; these compounds are present in most, if not all, commercial bread. But you should be aware that products lacking the "artificial preservative" calcium propionate are much more likely to become moldy.

Although food waste is a serious problem, it pales in light of the possible health dangers of reducing some other types of additives. If, for example, in an attempt to "go natural," nitrates and nitrites were left out of meat products, botulism toxin would again become a very real risk to life and health. This subject will be covered further in chapter 6.

FDA May Lower the Boom on Misleading Food Labeling

Taking full advantage of consumers' wish for healthful food, many manufacturers are labeling food products with misleading statements. Take the term "light," for example. Did you know that it has had no legal meaning? Or that it can refer to color, texture, odor, calories, weight, or sodium content. Or that choosing a "light" oil won't reduce your dietary fat or calorie content because all oils provide the same amount of fat and calories.

Honey Nut Cheerios contains more sugar than honey and far more salt than nuts. Stouffer's proudly advertises its *Lean Cuisine* dinners with the statement, "Never more than a gram of sodium." While the claim is true, the intended message is not. At present, there are countless other confusing—downright dishonest—label claims on food.

Two such questionably labeled foods made the headlines in mid-1991 when the FDA decided to crack down on food manufacturers dabbling in deceitful ditties. *Citrus Hill Fresh Choice* orange juice was the first to feel the squeeze. The FDA forced its manufacturer, Procter & Gamble, to remove the term "fresh" from the label of this product, which is actually made from concentrate. Ragu Foods was next in line; FDA officials similarly ordered them to remove the word "fresh" from their

Ragu Fresh Italian pasta sauces, which are heat-processed and not actually fresh. We do, however, question whether wholesome products like these should be occupying the limited time of FDA officials.

Congress encouraged the FDA to crack down on food labeling when it passed the Nutritional Labeling and Education Act in the fall of 1990. The unanimously passed law not only gives FDA more muscle to force food manufacturers to hawk their products honestly, but also requires straightforward nutrition labels for all foods, including fresh fruits and vegetables. The new nutrition labeling is intended to draw attention away from vitamin content (since very few Americans are deficient in most vitamins) and instead make it easier to determine the calorie, fat, and sodium content of foods. This will make it easier for people who must monitor their intake of these dietary constituents.

While Congress was considering passage of the Nutrition Labeling and Education Act, the FDA began proposing new labeling regulations. These would be the first changes in labeling requirements since the 1970s (except for sodium rules added in the 1980s). According to FDA Commissioner David A. Kessler, M.D., J.D., they were developed with a simple goal in mind:

> A label the public can understand and count on—that would bring them up-to-date with today's health concerns. It is a goal with three objectives: First, to clear up confusion; second, to help us make healthy choices; and third, to encourage product innovation, so that companies are more interested in tinkering with the food in the package, not the words on the label.

In November 1991 the FDA published sweeping proposals that could become final rules by November 8, 1992 and be required on all packaged foods by May 8, 1993. Unless there is a change or a delay, you'll find such newly labeled products on supermarket shelves in 1993. Here's a summary of some of the proposed rules:

1. *Nutrient content:* The required list of nutrient characteristics has been changed to reflect our nation's changing health concerns. The required items will be: total calories, calories derived from fat, total fat, saturated fat, cholesterol, total carbohydrates, complex carbohydrates, sugars, dietary fiber, protein, sodium, vitamins A and C, calcium, and iron. Because Americans generally don't suffer from deficiencies of the B vitamins thiamine, riboflavin, and niacin, listing them will become optional. Vitamin and mineral content will be listed as percentages of U.S. Reference Daily Intakes (RDI), a new system of values that reflects what people need more accurately than the previous U.S. RDA system. (Because most RDI values will be lower, the percentages of vitamins and minerals on most food labels will generally be higher than they have been in the past. Of course, the health food industry is worried that people will be less likely to take supplements if they think they are getting adequate nutrition from their normal eating patterns.)

2. *Serving sizes:* The new rules can help consumers better understand and be able to compare nutrition listings from product to product. Also, the serving-size listings must reflect the amount of that food that people actually eat. Finally, portion sizes will have to be listed in common household measurements, such as one cup, as well as in metric measures, such as 240 milliliters.

3. *Descriptive terms:* Terms such as "low," "reduced," and "diet" will describe calories, when the product modifications meet certain specifications. The terms "free," "low," "very low," and "reduced" must describe the level of sodium, according to certain specifications. The terms "high" and "source of"

will be defined as terms intended to emphasize the beneficial presence of certain nutrients. "High" can be used only when that food provides 20 percent or more of the RDI in a normal size serving. "Source of" will only be allowed when it provides 10 to 19 percent of the RDI. Other specifications have been proposed to make these terms more meaningful.

Definitions related to fat and cholesterol: Extensive reform in labeling terms relative to fat and cholesterol will be one of the most important changes. Not only are terms strictly defined, but all claims of cholesterol content will be prohibited when a food contains more than 2 grams of saturated fat per serving.

Other proposed reforms would restrict use of the word "fresh" to raw food, regulate nutrient claims for substitute foods, control the health claims that appear on food labels, label vitamin and mineral supplements more clearly, and bring about labeling of most raw produce and fish.

The Bottom Line

People who decide to go natural have to dedicate considerable money and time to this pursuit. Price markup is, by far, the healthiest thing about natural foods and products!

Why do they cost more? First, sellers are reaping the usual high profits associated with marketing specialty foods. Second, price is directly related to the fact that producing food grown "organically" just "naturally" costs more. That's because "organic" agricultural supplies cost more. Organic fertilizers cost from thirty to eighty times as much as commercial fertilizers. And crop losses are much greater when pesticides are not used.

It's difficult to estimate how much money your first visit to Healthfoodland may cost. The argument that "life comes from the sea" is not really a good reason for buying a big bottle of sea water. If you purchase sea salt without added iodide, a necessary nutrient, you may also be advised to buy kelp (which contains iodine) to supplement the salt you just paid more for because it was "natural" and iodide-free.

The price markup of everyday food items varies from place to place. Early in 1990 a survey of stores in Houston, Texas, yielded this comparison:

Food	Regular Section of Supermarket	Health Food Store
Unbleached white flour	$1.49 (5 lb)	$1.75 (2 lb)
Corn oil (1 qt)	2.36	4.47
Peanut oil	5.25 (2 qt)	7.17 (1 qt)
Salt, plain (26 oz)	.36	1.72
Apple cider vinegar (1 qt)	1.43	3.89
Oat bran cereal, hot (1 lb)	1.65	2.35
Spinach fettuccini	.63 (12 oz)	1.40 (8 oz)
Linguini	.95 (12 oz)	1.48 (8 oz)
Dill pickles (1 qt)	2.09	4.60
Molasses	2.29 (16 oz)	4.00 (15 oz)
Fruit spread, sweetened with fruit juice (10 oz)	1.89	2.29

Health food advocates would have to hold some pretty strong convictions to believe so-called natural foods are worth the significant price difference!

4

Beware! It's Natural

"One side will make you grow taller, and the
other side will make you grow shorter."
One side of what? The other side of what?
thought Alice to herself.
"Of the mushroom," said the Caterpillar.

—Lewis Carroll
Alice in Wonderland

Concern about "Chemicals"

The third cornerstone on which Healthfoodland is built is the
myth that natural is always better than artificial, or "be afraid of
anything that's hard to pronounce!"

Most people have little or no idea what is actually in the
"natural" foods and drinks they consume. If you were to ask a
couple of your friends to drop by for a cup of butyl, isoamyl,
phenyl ethyl, hexyl and benzyl alcohols, tannin, essential oils,
geraniol, and caffeine, they would probably have "made other
plans." However, if you merely invited them for a friendly cup
of tea, they might find their calendar was clear.

Underlying the natural foods movement is the mistaken idea
that "artificial" foods are made up of "chemicals," while natural
foods are "chemical-free." After all, who wants to snack on

63

mixtures of chemicals with names you can't even pronounce? Butylated hydroxyanisole (BHA) and butylated hydroxytoluene (BHT) . . . monosodium glutamate . . . xanthan gum. It's enough to make you wonder if you're eating anything that's wholesome!

Consumers' misconceptions are fed by journalists like Gerald Gold of *The New York Times,* whose early review of the egg substitute *Egg Beaters* said, "You would have to be a chemist to tell what you are really eating, even though all the products list their ingredients, for some of them are mostly chemicals." *Egg Beaters* does indeed contain a long list of chemicals: egg white, corn oil, nonfat dry milk, emulsifiers (vegetable lecithin, mono- and diglycerides, and propylene glycol monostearate), cellulose and xanthan gums, trisodium and triethyl citrate, artificial flavor, aluminum sulfate, iron phosphate, artificial color, thiamin, riboflavin, and vitamin D.

Someone even mildly anxious about chemicals might run, not walk, to the dairy case and pick up a dozen of the old reliables. But let's compare the "natural chemicals" in the everyday hen's egg: ovalbumin, livetin, sodium chloride, conalbumin, cholesterol, lutein, ovomucoid, lecithin, lipids, zeaxanthine, mucin, globulins, phosphates, amino acids, and lipovitellin. No, this list hasn't been adulterated by modern "henning" practices—even your great-grandmother packed away those natural chemicals with each egg she ate.

Just to be sure you get the point that "natural" and "organic" don't mean chemical-free, consider the chemicals in chilled melon and coffee. Melons contain starches, citric acid, vitamin A, sugars, succinic acid, riboflavin, cellulose, anisyl propionate, thiamin, pectin, amyl acetate, phosphates, malic acid, ascorbic acid. Coffee contains caffeine, dimethyl sulfide, butanol, essential oils, propionaldehyde, methylfuran, methanol, acetone, isoprene, acetaldehyde, methyl acetate, methylbutanol, methyl formate, furan, ethanol, diacetyl.

The bottom line is that every living thing, every animal and plant, is composed of chemicals—even the human body. We are, among other things, 65 percent oxygen, 18 percent carbon, 10 percent hydrogen, 3 percent nitrogen, 1.5 percent calcium, 1 percent phosphorus, with traces of silver, iron, and many other elements. This certainly doesn't make our bodies artificial instead of natural!

The Poisons in Your Health Foods

The back-to-nature enthusiasts operate under two major misconceptions. First, they believe that "natural" is synonymous with "chemical-free." Second, and more significant, they believe that "natural" means *danger-free*. To the contrary, scientists have long known that nature's horn of plenty has far more toxins and carcinogens than all "artificial" or synthetically produced foods combined. Take, for example, the traditional Thanksgiving meal. The American Council on Science and Health has listed the major toxins in each food. Here's the menu and some of the naturally-occurring toxins:

Appetizers

Cream of mushroom soup: Hydrazines
Carrots: Carotatoxin, myristicin, isoflavones, nitrate
Radishes: Glucosinolates, nitrate
Cherry tomatoes: Hydrogen peroxide, nitrate, quercetin glycoside, tomatine
Celery: Nitrate, psoralens
Assorted nuts: Aflatoxins

Entrees

Roast turkey: Heterocyclic amines, malonaldehyde

Bread stuffing (with onions, celery, black pepper, and mushrooms): Benzo(a)pyrene, di- and triethyl carbamate, furan derivatives, dihydrazines, psoralens, safrole

Cranberry sauce: Eugenol, furan derivatives

Choice of vegetable

Lima beans: Cyanogenetic glycosides

Broccoli spears: Allyl isothiocyanate, nitrate, glucosinolates, goitrin

Baked potato: Amylase inhibitors, arsenic, isoflavones, nitrate, oxalic acid, solanine, chaconine

Sweet potato: Cyanogenetic glycosides, furan derivatives, nitrate

Rolls: Amylase inhibitors, diacetyl, benzo(a)pyrene, ethyl carbamate, furan derivatives

Desserts

Pumpkin pie: Myristicin, nitrate, safrole

Apple pie: Acetaldehyde, isoflavones, phlorizin, quercetin glycoside, safrole

Beverages

Coffee: Benzo(a)pyrene, caffeine, chlorogenic acid, hydrogen peroxide, methylglyoxal, tannins

Tea: Benzo(a)pyrene, caffeine, quercetin glycosides, tannins

Red wine: Alcohol, ethyl carbamate, methylglyoxal, tannins, tyramine

Water: Nitrate

We could safely say that none of us worries that we'll be poisoned by Thanksgiving dinner (although we may legitimately worry about gaining a few pounds!). This Thanksgiving dinner menu, printed with the naturally occurring toxins, drives home a very important point, perhaps said best by the Renaissance physician Paracelsus: *Sola dosis facit venenum—it's the dose that makes the poison.* Little did Paracelsus know we would apply his adage to the very sustenance on our tables!

Consider the potential harm of some of these Thanksgiving poisons you're eating:

• Carotatoxin acts as a nerve poison in animals.

• Tomatine interferes with nerve transmission in humans.

• Malonaldehyde, furan derivatives, and many heterocyclic amines are mutagens in test systems. (A mutagen is a something that causes mutation, a permanent change, in a gene.)

• Allyl isothiocyanate, acetaldehyde, benzo(a)pyrene, ethyl carbamate, many hydrazines, and quercetin glycosides are carcinogens in animals.

Well, there's still your coffee. At least that should be good to the last drop. Isn't it? But, among other things, coffee contains caffeine. Caffeine, a "natural" substance found in many soft drinks, as well as coffee and tea, can have a number of harmful effects. In large amounts, or in sensitive individuals, caffeine can increase heart rate and cause irregular heartbeats in both healthy people and patients with heart disease. Doctors often advise pregnant women to limit caffeine since some animal studies suggest a link between this "natural" drug and birth defects. And parents of children who suffer from insomnia, rapid heartbeat, restlessness, and irritability are cautioned to check the child's intake of caffeine.

A fatal dose of caffeine, though, requires about ninety cups of coffee. Similarly, you would have to eat no less than 3.8 tons of turkey (at one sitting) to be poisoned by the naturally occurring malonaldehyde. Nor, of course do the cinnamon in apple pie or the black pepper in turkey stuffing pose a health threat. You would have to eat fifty pounds of cinnamon or black pepper to be threatened by cancer—though you'd most certainly sneeze yourself to death first!

No Shortage of Naturally Occurring Toxins

While most naturally occurring toxins are harmless at the everyday doses we generally consume, some do pose a real threat to health. To further illustrate our point that natural isn't always safer, *and* to warn you against potentially dangerous "health" and "organic" foods, we note the following:

• *Sassafras:* Safrole, a component of the natural sassafras plant and oil of sassafras, was used to flavor root beer until 1960. Although it fits the food faddists' definition of a purely natural substance, research studies proving that it caused liver cancer in some animals led the FDA to ban it as a food additive. In spite of this, sassafras made a comeback as a "health food" tea during the early 1970s—a period of rapid growth in the number of health food stores. FDA officials, who were understandably alarmed to find that fresh sassafras roots had become popular, acted quickly to remove them from the market. Now sassafras tea products can be sold only if the safrole has been removed.

• *Apricot kernels:* Another "purely natural" product that can have serious consequences is the apricot kernel. Unfortunately for the people who buy this product from their neighborhood health food store, apricot kernels contain "purely natural" hydrogen cyanide. Some people have died from cyanide poisoning after consuming apricot kernels.

• *"Porcupine fish":* Also known as fugu fish or balloon fish, this strange sea creature is a famous Japanese delicacy. However, a potent poison, tetradotoxin, is concentrated in its liver, ovaries, and the testes. Within minutes of eating just a small bit of toxic material from the balloon fish, a person experiences numbness of the lips, tongue, and fingertips. Death can quickly follow. The Japanese now license chefs who are formally trained in identifying and discarding the poisonous organs. Although the porcupine fish presents no problem when properly prepared, hundreds, if not thousands, of people throughout history have died from consuming its poison-containing organs. However, some Japanese men who know this still eat porcupine fish testes with the hope of enhancing virility—sometimes with fatal consequences.

• *Quail*: Eating this favorite game bird can also be risky. Pliny the Elder, Galen, Lucretius, and Avicenna all mention the dangers of eating quail. The quail's lethal nature may result from its eating of poisonous substances such as hemlock. Whatever the nature of the toxic substances, it appears that certain quail contain alkaloids that can be fatal if consumed by humans. In Algeria, where a so-called green quail is eaten, there are reports of people developing nausea, vomiting, shivers, and partial, slow-spreading paralysis—all associated with this fowl (but decidedly foul) delicacy.

• *Mushrooms:* Mushroom lovers should know that there are over twenty-five highly poisonous species of natural mushrooms. Perhaps the best known is the "death angel" variety, which produces rapid degeneration of the liver, kidney, heart, and muscles.

• *Bracken fern:* That tender and tasty sprout that looks a lot like asparagus may actually be bracken fern. Even after being cooked, this plant is a powerful cancer-causing agent. Cows feeding on bracken fern suffer damaged bone marrow and swollen membranes of the bladder. Health officials are concerned about this and other innocent-looking, unfamiliar vegetables, since "natural diners" may feel that it's safe to eat anything in the garden that looks tempting—a practice that can have serious and even fatal consequences.

• *Honey:* Honey is one of the most widely promoted health foods. But certain collections of honey can cause severe problems. Honey from certain geographical areas can become contaminated by substances that act as nerve and muscle poisons. This "mad honey," as it is called, occurs when bees carry nectar from certain rhododendron, azalea, and laurel species to their honey. A host of very uncomfortable symptoms occur minutes to hours after ingesting this honey: tingling and numbness of the extremities; a weakened, very slow pulse rate; loss of coordination; muscle weakness; and vomiting. Honey poisoning, though, is rarely fatal. Honey should not be fed to infants because their immature stomachs allow the botulism bacillus to multiply if it happens to be present. (Adults don't get the infant form of botulism because they can destroy the bacillus efficiently.)

Rebuking Technology Can Be Dangerous

"Organic farmers" who choose to grow food without agricultural chemicals may well expose themselves to dangerous natural toxins. Agricultural chemicals, without a doubt, have largely eliminated the threat of naturally growing fungi and microorganisms that can produce very poisonous "natural" substances. Consider the following examples:

• *Apple cider:* Apple cider presents an interesting problem. As we noted in chapter 1, the public became very alarmed about the presence of the growth-regulator Alar in apples and apple products in 1989. Alar causes all the apples on a tree to ripen at the same time for easier harvesting. Cider made from fallen apples that have become moldy may contain patulin, a poisonous metabolite shown to produce cancer. If unfermented apple cider is made from organically grown apples that have fallen to the ground and begun to rot, it could contain patulin. According to *Nutrition Reviews,* "Juice derived from apples grown on organic farms where trees have not been sprayed is likely to contain considerable quantities of fungus-rotten apple extract. This fact should be of concern to advocates of organic farming practice."

• *Peanuts and corn:* In 1960 thousands of turkeys died in England and other countries of what was temporarily called "turkey X disease." Soon afterward, it was learned that the deaths were due to natural aflatoxin molds (*Aspergillus flavus*) in the turkey food.

Molds that produce aflatoxin are widely distributed in air and soil and are able to grow on a variety of substances, including peanuts, rice, corn, soybeans, whole oats, wheat (particularly shredded wheat), figs, grain sorghum, cottonseed, and certain tree nuts. Aflatoxins are considered a natural poison and have been shown to produce liver cancer and genetic changes in experimental animals.

Considerable evidence suggests that aflatoxins in moldy peanut products may play a role in the development of human liver cancer. Studies of regions in Africa and southeast Asia have linked the prevalence of liver cancer to the level of aflatoxins occurring naturally in the local diet.

A 1969 study in the Philippines noted that a sample of locally manufactured natural peanut butter was highly contaminated with aflatoxins. And the FDA has acknowledged that small amounts of natural aflatoxins can be found in U.S. peanut products. A nationwide study of peanut butter conducted by the FDA in the 1970s found aflatoxins in one-fourth of the products but in amounts too small to cause illness in humans. Commercial peanut products sold in this country can have no more than five parts per billion—traces that can and often do remain in spite of cooking, processing, or home-roasting peanuts. (Again, though, be assured that this level does not threaten human health. We only use the example to make the point that something natural like peanut butter can have toxins—toxins that consumers normally ignore in their quest to eliminate "unnatural" products from their diet.)

Corn also can become contaminated with aflatoxins, especially in seasons following a drought. The FDA monitors corn products as well as milk and other dairy products from animals that might have been fed aflatoxin-contaminated corn.

• *Rye and wheat:* Ergotism ("St. Anthony's fire)" has been known for hundreds of years. This disease results from consuming ergot, an alkaloid-containing parasitic fungus that most frequently attacks rye fields in damp climates. The alkaloids are toxic, and some are related to the hallucinogen lysergic acid diethylamide (LSD). Because the alkaloids cause muscles and blood vessels to contract, ergot has long been used to treat migraine headaches, induce abortions, and stop bleeding after childbirth. In large doses, however, it can reduce circulation to the fingers and toes so severe that they become gangrenous. Diarrhea, colic, headaches, vomiting, and convulsions also can occur.

It's believed that in the year 944 more than forty thousand people died during an epidemic of ergot poisoning in Europe. But ergotism was not just an ancient threat: ergot poisoning remains a danger in the twentieth century. In 1951 there was an outbreak of "bread poisoning" in Southern France. Of the two hundred people who became ill after eating bread made from ergot-containing grain, twenty were classified as "temporarily insane," and four died. Although some scientists believe there might have been another substance in addition to ergot responsible for this incident, the results were undeniably dramatic. While some of the victims tried to fly off buildings, others screamed in terror because they believed they were surrounded by fire and under attack by prehistoric beasts.

In addition to causing "St. Anthony's fire," natural ergot has also been linked to tumor formation in certain laboratory animals. Be assured, however, that major bread industries in the United States routinely and carefully examine grain for ergot contamination.

• *Rice:* That old stand-by becomes potentially dangerous if it isn't fresh. Stored rice is easily contaminated by a number of fungi, especially *Penicillium* and *Aspergillus* species. When large amounts of this so-called "yellow rice" (not the same as rice seasoned with saffron) were given to rats and mice, the animals developed both cancerous and noncancerous tumors. Yellow rice has also caused human illness.

Actual vs. Theoretical Risks

As we hinted with our Thanksgiving menu, lots of foods contain chemicals that can cause trouble under some circumstances but not others. Here are actual or theoretical dangers posed by several more foods:

• *Spinach:* Popeye might bite his pipe in two if he heard some of the things we now know about his beloved spinach. Spinach, and several other vegetables, are our major source of naturally occurring nitrates. (Beets, radishes, eggplant, celery, lettuce, collards, and turnip greens also have relatively high amounts of nitrates.) Without a doubt, there are more nitrates in spinach and these other vegetables than in any cured meat you can eat.

Actually, it's not nitrates that are of concern, but a product that the body changes them to—nitrites. These nitrites then combine with certain organic substances (amines) to form nitrosamines, which have been linked to causing cancer. In most nitrate-containing vegetables, nitrates don't pose a threat to health because they usually aren't converted to nitrites. But if spinach is stored under conditions that allow microorganisms to grow, nitrates quickly change to nitrites in significant levels. In fact, cases of "spinach sickness" have been reported following a meal including fresh spinach that had been standing at room temperature for some time after cooking. Experts in food chemistry now recommend that home-prepared spinach never be stored for subsequent feeding. They also recommend that foods such as spinach and beets, which contain high levels of nitrate, should not be introduced into the diet of children below three months of age.

Do remember, though, that spinach is an excellent, nourishing food when it's eaten in moderation and is fresh. We only present this information to emphasize our point that "natural" does not always mean "without risk."

• *Sweet potatoes:* All is not sweet with the sweet potato. There are recorded cases of large-scale outbreaks of sweet potato poisoning among farm animals. Cattle who have munched on sweet potatoes seem especially prone to develop a fatal condition involving water in their lungs, which apparently leads to suffocation. Some store-bought moldy sweet potatoes contain toxins that don't disappear after the food is boiled or baked. The moral of this vegetable course is to be sure your produce is fresh.

• *Greens:* Salad isn't always a healthy treat. Eating very large amounts of some salad vegetables—particularly cabbage, cauliflower, turnips, mustard, and collard greens—can lead to the development of goiter in susceptible people since these "goitrins" contain a substance able to block the body's absorption of iodine.

• *Table salt:* We know that even simple table salt (sodium chloride) may cause problems if consumed in large amounts. Animal studies have shown that excess salt intake interferes with growth. In humans, congestive heart failure is worsened by high levels of salt intake, as are certain types of kidney diseases and high blood pressure.

• *Bananas:* A high incidence of right-sided heart lesions has been found in a group of Africans relying on bananas as their main food source.

• *Lima beans:* Don't let your kids get a hold of this feisty fact: Lima beans harbor tiny amounts of hydrogen cyanide. Again, however, even lima-bean devotees can't overdose on the deadly chemical. Perhaps by now, we're successfully driving home the point that "it's the dose that makes the poison."

• *Nutmeg:* A pinch of nutmeg will make your pumpkin pie scrumptious, but dipping into the nutmeg jar is guaranteed to affect you adversely. Nutmeg, the dried kernel of the seeds of the nutmeg tree, contains the hallucinogen myristicin. A nutmeg overdose can cause euphoria and hallucinations, accompanied by very unpleasant symptoms of abdominal pain, vomiting, insomnia, incoherence, depression, stupor, and possible liver damage.

• *Potatoes:* The common potato contains more than one hundred fifty known chemical substances. Included among them are solanine alkaloids, oxalic acid, arsenic, tannins, nitrate, and more than one hundred other items of no recognized nutritional value to humans. The potato's solanine is exactly the same substance found in the leaves of the deadly nightshade plant. Most of the solanine found in potatoes is near the skin, especially in the green portion that has been exposed to the sun or artificial light; such green-tinted skin should be discarded. Our average intake of over more than one hundred pounds of potatoes per year provides enough solanine to literally kill a horse. The critical distinction, however, is that we don't get enough of this chemical at any one time to threaten health; even potato skin lovers needn't forgo their habit.

• *Water:* Even water can be fatal at excessive doses. An unpleasant form of suicide practiced in some Oriental countries consists of drinking great quantities of water.

• *Wheat germ:* Although rich in protein, vitamins, and minerals, wheat germ is one of those marginally helpful and potentially harmful health foods. This stems from two points. First, one must consume large quantities of it to benefit from the nutrients (at the expense of many excess calories). Second, the fat in wheat germ spoils easily under improper storage conditions, rendering it rancid and susceptible to fungi.

• *Estrogen* is found in physiologically insignificant quantities in eggs, honey, carrots, soybeans, wheat, rice, oats, barley, potatoes, apples, cherries, plums, garlic, sage leaves, parsley, and licorice root.

• Traces of *arsenic* are found in many fruits, vegetables, cereal products, meats, dairy products, and various shellfish such as oysters and mussels. To be sure, this arsenic occurs naturally and is not due to environmental pollution. Although large doses will do you in, medical research suggests that humans need trace amounts for good health!

Well, What Can We Eat?

This discussion of toxins in naturally occurring substances isn't meant to alarm you. Rather, it's meant to illustrate the critical distinction between *potentially toxic* and *actually hazardous* substances. The great majority of these potentially toxic foods are not hazardous because the dose we ingest is so minuscule. *It's the dose that makes the poison.*

Beyond the dose issue, two other essential points explain why we don't become ill after eating perfectly "natural" foods every day.

First, individual chemicals don't appear to be additive. This means that the two or three different toxic substances present in tiny amounts in lima beans, potatoes, or any other food don't add up to create a hazard. Maintain an important distinction: Too much of *one* chemical substance (either from one food or a combination of foods) can indeed become hazardous.

Second, there's evidence that the toxicity of one element is often counteracted by the presence of an adequate amount of another. For example, the poisonous effects of cadmium in the diet are reduced by accompanying high levels of zinc. Mark Twain actually was correct to some extent when he said, "Part of the secret of success in life is to eat what you like and let the food fight it out inside."

This brings us back to the commonsense observation that the "safety in numbers" concept still holds true. A well-rounded diet that eliminates known hazards will contribute to, not undermine, health. Follow two rules: Be moderate about everything you eat. And don't get caught up in the false idea that "if it's natural it's got to be good for you."

5

The Great Supplement Scam

"Speak English!" said the Eaglet.
"I don't know the meaning of half those
long words, and, what's more, I don't
believe you do either!"

—Lewis Carroll
Alice in Wonderland

Too Much of a Good Thing

The fourth cornerstone of Healthfoodland rests on two mistaken ideas: that vitamins and other supplements work wonders, and that you aren't likely to get too much of them. Before discussing the problems with these premises, let's begin with a short course in vitamin and mineral basics.

Vitamins are organic (carbon-containing) substances needed by the body in *very tiny* amounts. Someone whose diet lacks a particular vitamin for a long period of time can develop a deficiency disease specific for that vitamin. The disease is cured by adding the vitamin back into the diet.

The vitamins needed by humans are A, C, D, E, K, and the eight B-complex vitamins: thiamin (B_1), riboflavin (B_2), niacin (B_3), pyridoxine (B_6), cobalamin (B_{12}), folic acid, biotin, and pantothenic acid. Vitamins A, D, E, and K are fat-soluble and are stored in the body's fat. The rest are water-soluble and are stored in limited amounts in the body's fluid stores.

Scientific experiments and case reports have indicated what levels of intake are needed to avoid vitamin deficiency diseases. To guide the planning of menus, these data have been used to develop the Recommended Dietary Allowances (RDAs). The RDAs are *not* minimums. To be on the safe side, they are based on the amounts needed to avoid deficiency plus generous additional amounts to allow for storage within the body. The RDAs for most vitamins are expressed in milligrams (mg): it takes a whopping 28,350 mg to make one ounce. The RDA for vitamin C is 60 mg per day—less than the amount in an 8-ounce glass of orange juice or a cup of broccoli.

Minerals are inorganic compounds, about twenty of which are considered essential for human health. The six that are needed in larger amounts (100 mg or more daily) are called major or macrominerals. The others, needed in smaller amounts, are called microminerals or "trace elements."

Crash course completed, let's move into murkier areas.

Phony "Vitamins" and "Supplements"

Many health faddists claim that other substances are vitamins. Two examples are "vitamin B_{15}" and "vitamin B_{17}." Neither of these, by any stretch of the imagination, is a vitamin! B_{15} products have been made with a variety of ingredients, some of which are carcinogenic. The FDA has ordered manufacturers to stop marketing B_{15}, but it is still available at health food stores. B_{17} was none other than laetrile, the notorious quack cancer remedy made from cyanide-containing apricot pits. Laetrile faded from the limelight after a U.S. Supreme Court decision upheld the FDA's efforts to stop its importation into the United

States, but it is still prescribed at a few Mexican clinics.

Rutin, bioflavonoids, inositol, and para-aminobenzoic acid (PABA) are also marketed as vitamins in Healthfoodland, even though none of them is essential for human health or serves any significant nutritional function when taken as a dietary supplement.

In ordinary use the term "dietary supplement" refers to any food substance or mixture of such substances consumed in addition to or in place of food. The most common supplements are vitamins and minerals. The scope of this term is much broader, however, in Healthfoodland. The variety of products sold as "supplements" (including many that contain no essential nutrients) is huge. Altogether, several hundred companies are marketing more than seven thousand such products. Garlic oil, bee pollen, and lecithin are just a few examples. Supplements are such big business that many health food stores make more money from selling them than they do from selling foods.

Vitamin Myths Abound

Over the years, many grossly inaccurate myths about vitamins and minerals have been widely circulated. For example:

• *If you stuff yourself with enough vitamins, minerals, and other supplements, you can negate the effects of poor health habits (such as overeating, undereating, smoking cigarettes, and not exercising).* Americans are notorious for wanting a quick way to fix what is wrong, especially without giving up what we enjoy.

• *If a little bit is good, then a lot must be a whole lot better.* Nothing could be further from the truth. The fact is that once the body has used the amounts of vitamins and minerals it needs, it doesn't need and can't use any more. (Liken this to a recipe that calls for pepper. If a little is good, you know from past experience that a lot *isn't* a whole lot better.) Vitamin overdosing can be very dangerous.

• *Supplements provide a way to attain "superhealth."* This set of myths is based mainly on misunderstanding and misusing facts. For example, a supplement misuser who knows that a certain vitamin is necessary for the nervous system to work properly may incorrectly conclude that a larger amount can overcome nervousness or improve memory. Very simply, the body just doesn't work this way! Think back to the recipe calling for pepper.

• *The body easily rids itself of excess vitamins.* Unfortunately, this isn't always true. Fat-soluble vitamins are not excreted efficiently. They are generally stored until they can be used up, and thus can accumulate to toxic levels. For example, excessive amounts of vitamin A can cause headache, increased pressure on the brain, bone pain, and damage to the liver. Excessive vitamin D can cause kidney damage. And high doses of vitamin E can cause fatigue and other problems.

The body stores water-soluble vitamins in modest amounts, with excesses excreted quickly in the urine. But large excesses of water-soluble vitamins can still cause trouble. High dosages of vitamin C can cause diarrhea and, if discontinued after months of use, can lead to "rebound" scurvy. Large doses of niacin can cause severe flushes, liver damage, and skin disorders. And megadoses of vitamin B_6 can damage the nervous system.

Help from the Mainstream

Several large pharmaceutical companies have helped popularize vitamins by promoting them with misleading ads. Several years ago, for example, E. R. Squibb & Sons, Inc., made the following claims in ads for its Theragran Stress Formula:

• Emotional stress increases the need for water-soluble vitamins.

• Smoking and ordinary physical activity increase the need for water-soluble vitamins in the amounts found in Squibb's so-called stress formula.

• People can't obtain the water-soluble vitamins lost as a result of nonsevere stress by eating a balanced diet, increasing food intake when necessary, or by taking an ordinary potency (100 percent RDA) multivitamin supplement.

• It is difficult to obtain biotin in an average diet. (This is untrue. Biotin deficiency occurs very rarely—in infants and in people eating large amounts of raw egg, which blocks its absorption.)

• People under emotional stress or ordinary physical stress are at risk for biotin deficiency.

• Taking Squibb's "stress formula" will reduce the effects of psychological stress.

In late 1985, faced with legal action by New York State Attorney General Robert Abrams, the company agreed to stop making these false claims. By 1989, however, they returned to their old tricks with misleading magazine and television ads suggesting that Theragran-M (a megavitamin supplement with added minerals) would make people more energetic. The company agreed to revise this commercial after consumer advocate Stephen Barrett, M. D., filed a complaint with the National Advertising Division (NAD) of the Council of Better Business Bureaus.

Squibb hasn't been the only large drug manufacturer involved in exaggerating the need for vitamins. From the mid-1970s through the mid-1980s, Lederle Laboratories advertised that "stress robs the body of nutrients" and suggested that its product Stresstabs would solve this supposed problem. Following action by Attorney General Abrams and criticism by *Consumer Reports* magazine, ads of this type were stopped.

During the mid-1980s, Hoffmann-La Roche advertised what it called "Protector Vitamins." Ads for these products stated that: (1) the cells of the body may be attacked by harmful chemical substances called free radicals that "may" contribute to the development of "certain chronic disease conditions"; (2) vitamins E, C, and beta-carotene (actually not a vitamin but a provitamin, which the body can turn into vitamin A) help protect cells from free-radical damage; and (3) these nutrients are available in common foods. The closing comment in the advertisement was: "If your diet, like that of so many people, is coming up short, consider taking Protector Vitamins E, C, and beta-carotene." Similar claims were made in a catalog of the AARP Pharmacy Service, the mail-order service for the American Association for Retired Persons.

The "Protector Vitamin" concept was based on a 1982 report by the National Academy of Sciences, which said that diets rich in certain nutrients are associated with a lower incidence of certain cancers. But the report also advised against taking supplements of these nutrients because it was not known which dietary components, if any, might be effective. The Roche/AARP ads implied just the opposite and greatly exaggerated the likelihood of dietary deficiency. After being challenged in complaints to NAD, the AARP Pharmacy Service said that advertising for "Protector Vitamins" would not be continued. Roche dropped the concept also, but has continued to hype beta-carotene. Its recent ads state that beta-carotene is being studied as a cancer preventive and that it is a good idea to include foods containing beta-carotene in your diet. (You can decide for yourself whether this information is provided as a public service or to stimulate the sale of beta-carotene supplements.)

Bad Advice in "Health Food" Stores

Mainstream advertising is just the tip of this fallacious-vitamin-advertising iceberg. "Health food" retailers and the manufacturers that supply them make wrong and sometimes dangerous claims about all sorts of "supplement" products. In its May 1985 cover story titled "Foods, Fads, or Frauds?" *Consumer Reports* magazine identified more than forty manufacturers who were marketing "supplement" products with claims that were illegal.

Although it is illegal for storekeepers to "diagnose" or "prescribe," it is common for them to do both. Investigators from the American Council on Science and Health demonstrated this in 1983 by making 105 inquiries at health food stores in a three-state area. Asked about eye symptoms characteristic of glaucoma, seventeen out of twenty-four salespeople suggested a wide variety of products for a person not seen; none recognized that urgent medical care was needed. Asked over the telephone about sudden, unexplained fifteen-pound weight loss in one month's time, nine out of seventeen recommended products sold in their store; only seven suggested medical evaluation. Seven out of ten stores carried "starch blockers" despite an FDA ban. Nine out of ten salespeople recommended bone meal and dolomite, products considered hazardous because of contamination with lead. Nine salespeople made false claims of effectiveness for bee pollen, and ten did so for RNA. The investigators concluded that most health food store clerks give advice that is irrational, unsafe, and illegal.

In 1989 volunteers of the Consumer Health Education

Council telephoned forty-one Houston-area health food stores and asked to speak with the person who provided nutritional advice. The callers explained that they had a brother with AIDS who was seeking an effective alternative treatment against the virus that causes it. The caller also explained that the brother's wife was still having sex with her husband and was seeking products that would reduce her risk of being infected, or make it impossible.

All forty-one retailers offered products they said could benefit the brother's immune system, improve the woman's immunity, and protect her against harm from the AIDS virus. The recommended products included vitamins (forty-one stores), vitamin C (thirty-eight stores), immune boosters (thirty-eight stores), coenzyme Q_{10} (twenty-six stores), germanium (twenty-six stores), lecithin (nineteen stores), ornithine and/or arginine (nine stores), gamma-linolenic acid (seven stores), raw glandulars (seven stores), hydrogen peroxide (five stores), homeopathic salts (five stores), Bach flower remedies (four stores), blue-green algae (four stores), cysteine (three stores), and herbal baths (two stores). Thirty retailers said they carried products that would cure AIDS. None recommended abstinence or use of a condom.

Fairy Tales about Specific Vitamins

Here is a small sampling of supplement fairy tales perpetuated by food faddists and well-meaning health advocates alike; we balance them with the true stories:

Fairy Tale #1: Vitamin E prevents and cures a great number of diseases. The true story is that vitamin E has no special preventive or curative power, and there is no reason at all for routine supplementation with vitamin E. When vitamin E first entered the spotlight, promoters claimed that it had all-but-magical powers. Large amounts of this "miracle worker in a capsule" were said to be useful in treating acne, atherosclerosis, cancer, cirrhosis of the liver, coronary heart disease (both preventing and curing heart attacks), diabetes, sexual frigidity, infertility, miscarriages, elevated cholesterol levels, muscular dystrophy, peptic ulcer, rheumatic fever, and blood clots. Even more fantastic, claimed the hawkers, it increased stamina and endurance as well as sexual potency (always an effective sales "hook"), improved sperm quality, and protected lungs from air pollution.

The one thing these claims for vitamin E have in common is that none of them is anchored in fact. Although vitamin E is necessary for health, supplements won't make you any healthier—unless, of course, you happen to be a white rat with a vitamin E deficiency. Many claims about vitamin E have been based on experiments in which vitamin E deficiencies were developed in laboratory animals. After it was found that fertility decreased in vitamin E-deficient rats, imaginative entrepreneurs began marketing vitamin E as a "potency" vitamin.

Vitamin E is so widely distributed in the foods we eat (vegetable oils, whole grains, and leafy vegetables) that no case of vitamin E deficiency due to dietary shortage has ever been reported in an adult American. Many vitamin E products contain forty to one hundred times the RDA, amounts that, when taken regularly, can cause fatigue and other adverse reactions.

Fairy Tale #2: Extra doses of vitamin A can contribute to strength and vitality. Without a doubt, excess vitamin A intake is harmful. Vitamin A poisoning can occur after taking 25,000 IU or more per day for several months. In addition, there's strong evidence that taking high doses of vitamin A during pregnancy can lead to birth defects. And yet, it's not uncommon for health faddists to recommend dosages of 25,000 IU or more per day.

Remember that well-balanced diets supply sufficient vitamin A for health. Remember, too, that the human body can store vitamin A, so that foods rich in vitamin A do not have to be eaten every day to ensure an adequate intake. Over a week or two, adults should take in the daily equivalent of 800 to 1,000 micrograms of retinol equivalent (RE). Each RE equals five International Units (IU) of vitamin A, an older measure still used on supplement labels.

Fairy Tale #3: High doses of vitamin C prevent colds and the flu. The roots of the vitamin C "controversy" are interesting. This heated debate began when Nobel Prize winner Linus Pauling claimed in his book *Vitamin C and the Common Cold* (1970) that massive doses of vitamin C would both prevent and cure the common cold. There was a flurry of interest in his ideas—and a great deal of professional criticism of his claims. The *American Journal of Public Health*, for example, stated:

> Professor Pauling would have been more prudent and would have rendered a greater public service had he presented his ideas to the scientific world for evaluation before recommending them to the public as a basis of action.

At least sixteen well-designed double-blind studies published in the scientific literature have failed to show that large doses of vitamin C are beneficial in preventing colds. Taking extra vitamin C once you have a cold may slightly lessen its symptoms, but the amount necessary to accomplish this can be obtained from drinking a few glasses of citrus fruit juice each day.

Just because vitamin C is water-soluble doesn't mean that taking a lot more than the RDA is harmless to health. Massive doses—the amounts Pauling recommends—can indeed have unpleasant and even dangerous side effects. They include diarrhea, kidney or bladder stones, and, in pregnant women, the risk of delivering babies susceptible to "rebound" scurvy (a withdrawal reaction when their overgenerous supply of vitamin C is cut off).

Fairy Tale #4: Because vitamin B_6 is water-soluble, it's safe to use large doses to treat premenstrual syndrome (PMS). There are actually two myths combined in this one fairy tale. First, there's no scientific evidence that megadoses of vitamin B_6 provide any relief for PMS sufferers. Second, doses of vitamin B_6 as low as 25 mg a day can cause neurological damage. (The 1989 RDA for vitamin B_6 is 1.6 to 2 mg/day for adults.)

In 1987 the medical journal *Acta Neurologica Scandinavia* reported that over one hundred women who had been taking large amounts of vitamin B_6 for more than six months suffered neurological abnormalities. Of the women who had higher than normal blood levels of B_6, 20 percent had been taking less than 50 mg per day, 38 percent had been taking at least 50 mg but less than 100 mg, 31 percent had been taking at least 100 mg but less than 200 mg, and 11 percent had taken at least 200 mg but less than 500 mg per day. These women experienced a variety of symptoms, including twitching, bone pain, abnormal skin sensations ("pins and needles," numbness, burning, crawling, and itching), and muscle weakness.

Fortunately, stopping high doses of vitamin B_6 soon enough reverses neurological symptoms. Continued high doses, however, can result in permanent neurological damage. Scientists don't know the minimum amount of vitamin B_6 that causes problems, but it's probably less than the dose commonly prescribed for treating PMS. Experts recommend B_6 supplementation only in verified cases of B_6 deficiency or when someone is taking a medication that interferes with normal B_6 metabolism.

Fairy Tale #5: If you take enough calcium, you won't develop osteoporosis. The true story is much more complicated.

The human body contains more calcium than any other mineral, and 99 percent of the body's calcium is stored in bone. Osteoporosis is a disease in which bones lose calcium, becoming more porous and fragile. When these weakened bones are subjected to pressure, they may break or collapse. One common result of osteoporosis is "dowager's hump"—the decreased height and stooped posture often seen in older women. It is also a common cause of hip fractures, especially in older women. It's estimated that osteoporosis afflicts one-fourth of women over age sixty.

Although osteoporosis itself isn't fatal, it causes an enormous amount of pain, disability, and financial loss, and can contribute indirectly to the death of women over age sixty. Hip fractures, for example, can have devastating consequences. Fewer than half the women who suffer a hip fracture regain normal function, and many die from the complications of confinement to bed, such as pneumonia or pulmonary embolism.

The "logic" behind the full-scale marketing of calcium supplements goes something like this: If osteoporosis is the result of too little calcium, you can prevent it by taking enough calcium. This sounds sensible enough, but the situation isn't that simple. All adults begin losing bone mass gradually after about age thirty-five. The hormone estrogen slows the absorption of calcium from bone, thereby protecting women from calcium and bone loss until they reach menopause. Once there's less estrogen available, calcium is removed from bones at a faster rate.

An adequate intake of calcium throughout life is an important factor in minimizing bone loss. However, sales promotions suggesting that taking large doses of this mineral is all that is necessary to prevent osteoporosis are a gross oversimplification. Other risk factors for the development of osteoporosis include a deficiency of vitamin D, which is important in calcium metabolism, lack of the mineral nutrient fluoride (another plus for fluoridated water), cigarette smoking, and lack of weight-bearing exercise. It would be difficult for anyone drinking a couple of glasses of milk each day to have a vitamin D deficiency, since milk is fortified with this vitamin. If you can't (or don't) drink milk, you can get the necessary vitamin D from a supplement. Be aware, however, that overdosing on D is as harmful as not having enough of it.

Despite these facts, sales of calcium supplements have been brisk. According to a study conducted by Business Communications Company, Inc., a Connecticut-based marketing research firm, sales of calcium supplements grew from $18 million in 1980 to about $240 million in 1986. And they continue to grow.

Finally, be advised that some calcium supplements sold in health food stores have proved unsafe. Products made from dolomite or bone meal may contain lead and can be harmful to health.

Fairy Tale #6: Lecithin is nature's protection against heart attacks. There is no evidence that dietary lecithin protects against heart attacks. In addition, the body manufactures its own. Lecithin is also used commercially as an emulsifier in various foods (see chapter 6). Since lecithin is naturally present in the body and is also added to the food supply, supplements are neither necessary nor helpful. Food faddists, however, have long claimed that lecithin cures arthritis, high blood pressure, and gallbladder problems, *and* improves memory and brain power. Other self-styled "experts" recommend using lecithin together with cider vinegar, kelp, and vitamin B$_6$ for rapid weight loss. But lecithin's primary selling point is the claim that it wards off heart disease. The faddists theorize that lecithin breaks up and scatters cholesterol in the blood so that it can't become attached to artery walls. Alas, a review of no less than twenty-four studies on lecithin and cholesterol published in the *American Journal of Clinical Nutrition* in 1989 concluded that lecithin does *not* reduce blood cholesterol levels or prevent atherosclerosis.

Fairy Tale #7: Large doses of the amino acid L-tryptophan are useful for treating insomnia, premenstrual syndrome, depression, stress, and drug and alcohol addiction. L-tryptophan is an essential amino acid, one that the body cannot produce internally. The required amounts are readily available from the protein foods in a balanced diet. During the late 1970s and early 1980s, L-tryptophan supplements grew rapidly in popularity, although they were never approved by the FDA for any use. Dr. Stephen Barrett has collected evidence that at least twenty-six companies made illegal therapeutic claims for L-tryptophan products in their ads, catalogs, and/or product literature. In addition, L-tryptophan was popularized through articles in books, "health food" magazines, and other literature.

Late in 1989 the United States Centers for Disease Control (CDC) announced that an epidemic of eosinophilia-myalgia syndrome (EMS) had begun. This is a devastating disease whose symptoms can include severe weakness, muscle and joint pain, swelling of the arms and legs, rash, fever, paralysis, and an abnormally high number of eosinophils (a type of white blood cell) in the blood. By mid-1991, more than fifteen hundred cases and about thirty deaths had been reported. Some people had become ill on doses in the range of 1,000 to 2,000 mg per day, but others had consumed less than 100 mg per day. Based on the suspected connection to L-tryptophan supplements, the FDA banned L-tryptophan products from the American marketplace.

The cause of the EMS epidemic was finally traced to L-tryptophan made by a single Japanese bulk supplier who had used a new manufacturing process. The process apparently introduced a dangerous contaminant that caused many users to become ill. However, the FDA has not ruled out the possibility that EMS may be associated with consumption of L-tryptophan itself or that some people are unable to metabolize it. In addition, a few cases of EMS have been reported in people who took supplements of the amino acid lysine.

Beyond the Myths: the Frauds these Myths Empower

Nine of the top ten health frauds reported by the *FDA Consumer* in 1989 involve nutritional supplements:

1. *Fraudulent arthritis cures*. These range from snake and bee venom, megadoses of vitamins, and Chinese herbal remedies to copper bracelets. It's estimated that 95 percent of the forty million Americans with arthritis try such "cures" at one time or another.

2. *Spurious cancer clinics*. Located mainly in Mexico, these offer unproven and ineffective treatments such as laetrile or vitamins and minerals. Their false promises are more serious than their inability to effect a cure. Some people who seek these "miracle" cures neglect proven treatment, often at the expense of their life.

3. *Bogus AIDS cures*. As yet, there is no cure for AIDS. Anything claimed to be one, then, should be immediately doubted. As is the case with cancer, AIDS patients should choose only approved and recommended therapies, which have

more potential to offer them survival until a cure *is* discovered.

4. *Instant weight-loss schemes.* (These might more accurately be called instant money-making schemes.) Overweight is a problem for one fourth of Americans, many of whom crave immediate results. Realizing this, many entrepreneurs offer gimmicks promised to provide easy weight loss. Grapefruit and fiber pills are just two examples.

5. *Fraudulent sexual aids.* These include products to enhance pleasure or cure impotence or frigidity. The FDA has concluded that no over-the-counter drug is safe and effective for this purpose and has banned the sale of such products. Some purported "aphrodisiacs" contain harmful ingredients.

6. *Quack baldness remedies and other appearance modifiers.* Entrepreneurs make millions of dollars by persuading people to buy their particular versions of the fountain of youth, including hair growers, wrinkle-removers, and bust developers. The only product approved for treatment of one particular type of baldness is the prescription drug Rogaine (minoxidil). The FDA banned the marketing of creams, lotions, and other external products with claims that they can grow hair or prevent baldness.

All bust developers are fakes. Most are gadgets or creams, but one imaginative product sold years ago was a protein supplement said to exert its effects in just the "right places."

7. *False nutritional schemes.* All sorts of food products are promoted as sure-fire cures for various diseases and conditions. Bee pollen, for example, is supposed to improve athletic performance, retard aging, promote weight loss, and relieve allergies (to list just a few of the claims). None of these claims has been proved. Worse yet, scientists do know that bee pollen is poten-

tially dangerous to someone with allergies, gout, or kidney problems (facts that bee pollen promoters may not bother to tell you).

8. *Chelation therapy.* Promoters of this treatment claim that intravenous infusions of a synthetic amino acid (EDTA) along with vitamins and minerals will clean out atherosclerotic plaque from the arteries and thereby prevent heart attack, circulatory disease, angina (chest pain), and strokes. Chelation therapy is often described as an effective alternative to coronary bypass surgery—which it is not. According to the FDA, people who shell out thousands of dollars for chelation therapy not only pay for an unproven treatment, but place themselves at risk for kidney disease, bone marrow depression, and convulsions. [Note: A controlled trial whose protocol was approved by the FDA was begun about two years ago to test whether chelation therapy is effective against intermittent claudication, a condition in which impaired circulation to the legs causes pain when the person walks. Chelation proponents have been trumpeting the very existence of the test as evidence that there is something to their claims. Although the trial should have been completed by now, no results have been publicly reported. Meanwhile, a Danish study found that chelation therapy was no more effective than a placebo against intermittent claudication.]

9. *"Candidiasis hypersensitivity" cures.* This alleged condition—sometimes referred to as "yeast infection"—is based on the notion that 30 percent of Americans suffer from multiple symptoms because they are allergic to a fungus normally present in warm, moist areas of the body. People who diagnose this "disease" (anyone from licensed medical doctors to health food faddists) claim that it causes fatigue, constipation, depression, anxiety, mental confusion, infertility, impotence, men-

strual problems, and a long list of other common symptoms.

People with lowered resistance (because of disease or anti-biotic medication) can develop a real yeast infection (candidiasis), but there is no evidence linking real candidiasis to the above laundry list of symptoms. The American Academy of Allergy and Immunology has labeled the concept of "candidiasis hypersensitivity" as "speculative and unproven," which is a polite way of stating that it is utter nonsense.

Who Takes Supplements?

If you're one of those Americans who doesn't use supplemental vitamins and minerals, you may wonder what all the fuss is about. You may indeed be surprised to learn what some recent surveys reveal about supplement usage:

• At least 36 percent, and possibly as many as 54 percent, of adults take one or more supplements.

• About 43 percent of children ages 2 to 6 take supplements.

• Among those who use supplements, 53.4 percent consume just one supplement, while 10.9 percent use from five to fourteen separate products *daily*.

• Supplement usage results in a wide range of vitamin and mineral intake, commonly from ten to fifty times the RDA for individual nutrients.

• More women than men in all age groups use supplements.

• The most widely used supplement is vitamin C (90.6 percent of supplement users take vitamin C), either alone or in combination with other nutrients.

• There are significant differences in supplement usage

between races—for both sexes, and in all age groups. The greatest difference is in people age sixty-five or older: 40 percent of whites and Hispanics but only 14 percent of blacks in this age category use supplements.

• Supplement use varies with family income: in families earning $40,000 per year or more, half of the children take supplements; only 23 percent of children in families with an income of less than $7,000 per year take them.

A 1987 report on adolescent beliefs about vitamin supplements was most interesting. Eighty-six percent of these fourteen- to eighteen-year-olds reported using vitamin/mineral supplements, offering the following common reasons for taking them:

"They make me healthy." (45 percent)
"My doctor tells me to take them." (39 percent)
"They help give me energy." (38 percent)
"They help cure my colds." (31 percent)
"They help my complexion." (29 percent)
"I don't eat right." (25 percent)
"They help me do better in sports." (23 percent)

Ironically, these surveys reveal that supplement users tend to have diets richer in many nutrients than their non-using counterparts! Equally ironic is the fact that people who use supplements often fail to choose the appropriate ones to compensate for the nutrients that may be lacking in their diet.

Does Anyone Need Supplements?
What the Experts Say

The prevailing opinion of medical and nutrition experts about supplements is best summarized in *Diet and Health,* a 765-page book issued by the National Research Council in 1989. One theme of this report could be described as "Vitamin Supplements: Try None a Day." Indeed, experts believe that few people need supplements. Some of the exceptions to this rule are:

• Women with excessive menstrual bleeding, who may need to take iron supplements.

• Women who are pregnant or breastfeeding, who need more of certain nutrients, especially iron, folic acid, and calcium.

• People with very low caloric intake whose diet does not meet their needs for most nutrients.

• Some vegetarians, who may not be receiving adequate vitamin B_{12}, calcium, iron, zinc, and protein quality.

• Newborns, who may need a single dose of vitamin K to prevent abnormal bleeding. This, of course, is done under the supervision of a physician.

• People with certain diseases and/or who take selected medications either or both of which can interfere with nutrient intake, digestion, absorption, or metabolism.

Separating Fact from Fiction

How can you tell when you are dealing with accurate health information or are being fed a "line" full of errors and lies? One good rule of thumb is to follow the wise old saying: if it sounds too good to be true, it probably is! Consumer activists Stephen Barrett, M.D. and Victor Herbert, M.D., J.D., suggest the following "red lights" to warn you that you're probably dealing with a health "quack":

• They use anecdotes and testimonials from satisfied customers to support their claims.

• They promise quick, dramatic, miraculous cures or claim that their product is based on a "secret formula" available only from this one company.

• They use disclaimers couched in pseudomedical jargon— offering to "detoxify" your body, to "balance" its chemistry, or to "strengthen" or "support" its various organs.

• They display credentials not recognized by responsible scientists or educators.

• They encourage patients to lend political support to their treatment methods. (This differs from the behavior of scientists who know that the way to establish the validity of a method is to conduct well-designed studies and report them in scientific journals.)

• They say that most disease is due to faulty diet and can be treated with "nutritional" methods.

• They recommend a wide variety of substances (such as ground-up animal organs) similar to those found in your body.

• When talking about nutrients, they tell only part of the story. They list all the horrible things that can happen if you don't get enough nutrients, but they neglect to mention that a balanced diet can provide the nutrients you need.

• They claim that most Americans are poorly nourished.

• They recommend that everybody take vitamins and/or health foods.

• They claim that modern processing methods and storage remove all nutritive value from our food.

• They claim that soil depletion and use of "chemical" fertilizers result in less nourishing food.

• They claim that under ordinary stress, and in certain diseases, your need for nutrients is increased to the point that dietary supplements are needed.

• They claim that you're in danger of being "poisoned" by food additives and preservatives.

• They claim that "natural" vitamins are better than "synthetic" ones.

• They claim that sugar is a deadly poison.

• They claim that fluoridation is dangerous.

• They recommend hair analysis for everyone as a method of detecting nutritional problems.

• They use a computer-scored questionnaire for diagnosing "nutrient deficiencies." (The computer, of course, is programmed to recommend supplements for everyone.)

• They tell you that it's easy to lose weight.

• They say not to trust your doctor and that most doctors are "butchers."

• They claim they are being persecuted by orthodox medicine, which, along with the government, is suppressing their wonderful discovery because it's controversial.

• They push you to buy a water purifier.

• Their treatment is promoted only in the back pages of magazines, over the phone, by mail-order, in newspaper ads made to look like news stories, or in 30-minute television commercials made to look like talk shows.

Wolves in Sheep's Clothing

It also pays to be wary if people whom you would otherwise trust tell you about wonderful results they have experienced by taking "nutritional" products they happen to be selling. Dozens of "multilevel" companies are marketing vitamins, herbs, diet formulas, and various other health-related items through person-to-person contact.

The name "multilevel" refers to the fact that these companies encourage their distributors to enlist more distributors who, in turn, sponsor additional distributors. When enough distributors have been recruited, the recruiters become eligible for bonuses based on their sales. Some multilevel companies, such as Shaklee Corporation and Amway Corporation, promote relatively expensive vitamin products as insurance against a faulty diet. Other companies, including Sunrider International and Nature's Sunshine Products, market herbal products with claims that they can prevent or treat various diseases.

Perhaps the most notorious multilevel company of recent times was United Sciences of America (USA), Inc., which began selling its wares at the beginning of 1986 and reached a sales volume of $10 million by its sixth month of operation. The company's main product was Master Formula, a concoction whose thirty-six ingredients included above-RDA amounts of several vitamins. The company's other products were: Formula Plus, a marine lipid concentrate rich in omega-3 fatty acids; Fiber Energy Bar, containing nine grams of fiber; and Calorie Control Formula, a high-fiber protein powder mix for use as a meal substitute.

What set USA apart was the claim that its dietary supplements had been developed by a prominent Scientific Advisory Committee that included two Nobel Prize winners. The products were marketed with a slick videotape, narrated by William

Shatner (Captain Kirk of "Star Trek"), that included scenes of a rocket launching, a giant computer bank, scientific laboratories, prominent medical institutions, and medical journals. During the tape, Shatner alleged that "our food, water, and air are becoming contaminated" by chemicals ("toxic killers"), that cancer is on the rise, that our soil is being depleted of "vital, life-giving nutrients and important earth minerals," that one out of every three families will be stricken with some form of cancer, and that two out of five people will die of heart disease or stroke. Then he described how the company's founder had developed a "brain trust of medical and scientific experts . . . to develop a complete nutritional program to protect us from the growing dangers that are threatening the health of our nation." Shatner also suggested that investing in USA's program would result in "looking your best, feeling maximum physical energy and mental well-being, enjoying total health."

The disease-related claims in the videotape made the products drugs subject to FDA regulation. Since the claims were false, they violated state laws as well. After scientific journals published several critical articles about USA, including two by Dr. Fredrick J. Stare, most of the scientific advisory committee resigned, sales slumped, and the company declared bankruptcy. A stern letter from the FDA and regulatory actions by authorities in Texas, New York, and California then stopped the company dead in its tracks, and it was liquidated in May 1987.

The FDA and "Vitamin Wars"

The FDA's current position on vitamin regulation dates to the early 1970s when it proposed new regulations for the nutrition labeling for food products. The proposal called for product labels to list ingredients, nutrient content, and other information in a standard format. This proposal was adopted without opposition. But the FDA also wanted to ban several claims related to the cornerstones of Healthfoodland. The proposed regulation would have banned label information that stated or implied that: (1) a food can prevent, cure, lessen, or treat any disease or symptom; (2) a balanced diet made up of ordinary foods can't supply adequate amounts of nutrients; (3) the daily diet may be inadequate or deficient due to food that is less nutritious because of the soil in which it is grown; (4) storage, transportation, processing, or cooking of a food is or may be responsible for nutritional inadequacy or deficiency in the daily diet; or (5) a natural vitamin is better than an added or synthetic vitamin. In addition, nutrients (such as rutin and bioflavonoids) that are not essential and have no known value for humans could not have been listed on the label.

Alarmed by these proposed rules, the health food industry mounted an extensive campaign to weaken the FDA's enforcement authority over vitamin products. Crying "Fight for your freedom to take vitamins!" the industry mobilized its members and many of their customers. Numerous articles supporting anti-FDA legislation appeared in health food magazines and chiropractic journals. Letter-writing kits were distributed through health food stores and multilevel distributors. The response to this campaign was so vigorous that several congressional representatives reported that they had received more mail about vitamins than about Watergate. In 1976, in response to this pressure, Congress passed the Proxmire Amendment to the Federal Food, Drug, and Cosmetic Act. This legislation prevents the FDA from regulating the dosage of dietary supplements unless it can be shown that they are inherently dangerous or are being marketed with illegal claims that they can prevent or treat disease.

The Proxmire Amendment, which one FDA Commissioner

called "a charlatan's dream," has made it difficult for the agency to ban "supplement" products that are worthless but not dangerous. It also has made some FDA officials reluctant to attack health food industry propaganda head-on. Enforcement actions were still taken against individual manufacturers who made illegal therapeutic claims for their products, but these actions stopped only a small percentage of illegal promotions.

In 1990 in response to public interest in clearer and more complete nutrition information on food labels, Congress passed the Nutrition Labeling and Education Act to increase FDA's authority and require new rules for nutrition labeling. Before the law was passed, however, the health food industry succeeded in exempting "dietary supplements of vitamins, minerals, herbs or other similar nutrients" from certain provisions applicable to foods. Instead, the law called for separate standards, which the industry hoped would be more lenient than those for foods.

David Kessler, M.D., J.D., who became FDA Commissioner in 1990, has a passionate interest in consumer protection. In response to the 1990 law, he set up an FDA task force to explore how dietary supplements should be defined, whether they should be regulated differently from foods and drugs, and whether additional laws are needed for the FDA to do the job. Noting that attempts by the FDA to regulate supplement products had had only limited success, he asked the task force to consider the best way for the agency to protect the public.

Fearing that the FDA will seek to ban or greatly restrict the sale of individual amino acids, herbal concentrates, and high-dose vitamin and mineral supplements, the health food industry has again sprung into action. Early in 1992 it began another campaign to flood Congress with letters urging it to curb the FDA's authority still further. As it did in the 1970s, the industry is defining the issue as "big government threatening to take away the right of individuals to obtain health products that they believe are important." What the industry really wants, however, is the right to continue to extract money from people who fall for its propaganda.

Consumer protection advocates want the Proxmire Amendment repealed so that the FDA can rid the marketplace of worthless "supplement" products. The "health food" industry wants the amendment strengthened to prevent effective FDA regulation. It remains to be seen whether Congress can ignore the industry's current campaign and do what is needed to protect the public.

6

What Have Additives Done for You Lately?

"Maybe it's always pepper that makes people hot-tempered," she went on . . . "and vinegar that makes them sour—and chamomile that makes them bitter—and barley sugar and such things that make children sweet-tempered."

—Lewis Carroll
Alice in Wonderland

Food for Thought

How nice it is to come home after a hard day's work and choose exactly what your palate craves from a well-stocked pantry and refrigerator—especially something that requires little or no preparation. However, quick-to-fix food must look attractive, have an enticing aroma, taste delicious, *and* be wholesome and nutritious.

It wasn't always that way in this country, and, in developing regions of the world, it still isn't that way. Throughout history, the amount and variety of foods available have been severely limited by such harsh realities as the changing seasons, poor weather, and food contamination. When there was enough food, it often provided a boring menu that took hours to prepare.

Food additives play a major role in making our food attractive, safe, enjoyable, varied, plentiful, nourishing, and easy to prepare. Unfortunately, however, additives are often misunderstood and are an object of fear and criticism.

The Earliest Food Additives

Let's look back for a moment. People today are hardly the first eaters to think about food additives and how they can make eating more enjoyable and predictable. Food additives have been around for a long time.

Around 300 B.C., Epicurus wrote of the joys of preserved cheese. Food colors were used in ancient Egypt. Kerosene was burned in ancient China to ripen bananas and peas. (This method worked because burning kerosene produced the ripening agents ethylene and propylene, names that are familiar today.) Back in 20 B.C., Horace described food that would last for at least a year as "the ultimate state of happiness." And Marco Polo, Christopher Columbus, Hernando Cortés, and many others were sufficiently enthusiastic about food additives to take the tremendous risks of ocean voyages to distant parts of the world. Marco Polo and Columbus sought spices to preserve foods and to make unexciting food more appetizing. For Columbus, discovery of the "New World" actually spelled failure for his original mission of establishing a shorter trade route between Europe and Asia for spices and other luxuries. Cortés sought the vanilla bean, an additive that made sixteenth-century food worth eating.

In 1691 an ambitious young businessman took out a patent for a method of "preserving by liquors or otherwise." In 1783 another entrepreneur obtained a patent for preserving salmon with spices. From their beginning, additives were intended to make food safer and tastier and daily life easier.

Today's additives go far beyond preserving cheese and salmon and offering vanilla flavor.

What Additives Add to Your Life

"Additives" are substances intentionally added to food to improve its appearance, taste, structure, storage life, safety, or nutritional value. These "direct additives" must be included on labels of meat and poultry products. Indirect additives, normally present only in trace amounts, result from contact between the food and agricultural chemicals, processing aids or equipment, and packaging. Contaminants, on the other hand, are substances in food, either present by accident or introduced during growth or processing, that are undesirable or potentially dangerous to consumers.

Many chemicals occur naturally in our foods (mentioned in chapter 4). It is easy for consumers to confuse these naturally occurring food chemicals with the chemicals that are added to foods. Using this alternate definition of food additive is thus helpful: "a pure substance of known composition that is added to food."

Critics often claim that food additives offer only slight benefit—that most additives are used purely to improve the appearance of food and that many involve outright trickery. A closer look at the role additives play will reveal that these "alarmists" fail to mention important facts.

Food Colors

Food colors are one type of additive that critics feel is unnecessary. Natural food enthusiasts claim not to care if their favorite fruit juice is passionate purple or bile green. Of course, that's their right—and there's no objection to the availability of color-additive-free products for such people. But there is another side to this "colorful" issue.

How would you like to eat a bowl of purple peaches with orange cream? Or some crispy toast with red butter and a tall glass of chilled green milk to wash it down? It doesn't sound too appetizing, does it?

A chef at a national convention for food color producers decided to try just such an experiment. He colored ordinary food products with the most unexpected colors. For example, the apple pie was a beautiful lilac and was elegantly dotted with black whipped cream. Many of his test subjects lost their appetite. The chef had demonstrated an important point: We "taste with our eyes." We may enjoy the unusual appearance of shamrock icing or green beer on St. Patrick's Day or the combination of black and orange food on Halloween. However, most of the time we like our food to look "the way it should." The way we expect a food to look tends to reinforce its taste.

Critics of food colors respond that we've been conditioned to want our foods to look a certain way. They argue that if canned cherries and other fruits were always a drab beige, we wouldn't miss the bright red we associate with maraschino cherries, and that if we were to stop using all food colors now, our children would grow up not knowing the difference.

These critics are ignoring the simple fact that food must be appealing to be eaten. This isn't the result of conditioning—it's what might appropriately be called a "gut reaction." Most shoppers, for example, will reject oranges with green-tinted peels even though they are assured the fruit is deliciously ripe. Butter normally has great variation in color, based on the season and the locality where it's produced. Shoppers are apt to return a stick of butter that is too pale for fear it is spoiled. The addition of food color assures a uniform color all the time.

When oleomargarine was introduced, it was illegal for manufacturers to add yellow coloring, because consumers might confuse it with butter. Later, oleo manufacturers were allowed to include a little packet of dye with their product. The great majority of buyers faithfully mixed this coloring into the white mass to make it more appealing.

Where Do Those Colors Come From?

There are three types of food colors: (1) those naturally present in foods, (2) those of natural origin that are added to foods, and (3) those manufactured in the laboratory. Nature obviously contributes to a wide range of food colors. For example:

• Chlorophyll is a green coloring matter extracted from plants.

• Anthocyanins, which range from blue to red, are found in flowers and plants.

• Carotenes, which are found in carrots, orange juice, apricots, and other foods, are used to give both oleomargarine and butter their golden yellow color.

• Saffron is made from the orange-colored aromatic dried stigmas (pollen-producing parts) of an old-world species of the iris family.

• Turmeric is made from the underground stem of a tropical plant of the ginger family.

• Annatto ("natural orange") is an extract obtained from the pulp around the seed of a small tropical tree.

• Cochineal is a natural red color made from the dried body of a female insect that grows on a type of cactus found in tropical and subtropical America.

Despite this interesting list, there just aren't enough natural food colors to meet the tremendous demand. Since the mid-1800s, food manufacturers have turned to the laboratory for more color options. Early research by the food dye industry focused on various by-products of coal, leading to the term "coal tar" dye. Although many other base substances are used to produce dyes today, the term "coal tar" is often used for all synthetically manufactured food colors. Food technologists produce pure dyes that resemble their natural counterparts so closely that it is virtually impossible to distinguish between the two.

Unlike coloring agents from "natural" sources, synthetic dyes require certification. This means that each batch of dye must be inspected and approved as it comes from the manufacturer before it can be used in food. In 1960, when enforcement of the Delaney Clause (discussed in chapters 7 and 8) began, there were about two hundred dyes in use. Since then these dyes have been undergoing testing to place them in one of three categories: (1) approved for certain specified uses (although still subject to review and further testing), (2) banned, or (3) provisionally approved for specific uses while testing continues.

The most widely used food coloring used to be amaranth, better known as FD&C Red No. 2. It was used in soft drinks, ice cream, baked goods, candy, and other foods. It had been used extensively in the U.S. since the turn of the century without any reported harm to human health. Despite this long history of safe use, Red No. 2 was called into question in 1972 after Russian scientists suggested that it might cause cancer or other health problems in animals. American researchers had difficulty evaluating these studies because the relative purity of Russian Red No. 2 wasn't known. But damaging doubts had been raised. The FDA spent two years doing additional intensive testing on Red No. 2 and again concluded that it was safe for use in human food. As described at that time by *Food Chemical News,* the "tests of Red No. 2 for carcinogenicity boiled down to two categories: one positive test and dozens of negative tests."

Although Red No. 2 had been tested more extensively than any other food coloring agent, some consumer activists still complained. Its tongue-twisting name (trisodium salt of 1-[4 sulfo-1-naphthylazo]-2-naphthol-3,6-disulfonic acid) made Red No. 2 a natural target for anyone suffering from "chemical phobia." In 1976, the prevailing fear of cancer won out and Red No. 2 was banned. Then, as now, the law didn't require proof that a dye was unsafe for humans. (FD&C Red No. 3 has also come under the FDA's regulatory scrutiny; see chapter 8 for a full discussion.)

Feingold's Theory of Hyperactivity

In 1973 the late Dr. Benjamin F. Feingold (then Chief of Allergy at San Francisco's Kaiser-Permanente Medical Center) presented his notion that food additives are a major cause of hyperactivity in children. Hyperactivity, now commonly called attention deficit disorder (ADD), is characterized by overactivity, impulsive behavior, short attention span, and learning problems. The accusations he made about coloring and flavoring agents in his book, *Why Your Child is Hyperactive,* were further popularized on television and radio talk shows. Numerous controlled research trials failed to verify Dr. Feingold's claims.

Nonetheless, Feingold was convincing enough to develop a faithful and vocal following of parents who believe the Feingold diet helps their hyperactive child. The result: this controversy has survived into the decade of the '90s.

Preservatives

> A wonderful bird is the pelican.
> His bill can hold more than his belican.
> He can take in his beak food enough for a week.
> But I'm damned if I can see how the helican.
>
> —Dixon Lanier Merritt

Unlike Mr. Merritt's pelican, humans need to eat every day. Our early ancestors spent much of their day foraging, tracking, and then preparing their sustenance. But today's life-style expects and demands a readily (if not immediately) available food supply.

Home refrigeration and commercial food preservatives have granted this wish. Except for a few highly perishable items, it is possible to obtain safe and wholesome food without shopping more than once a week. But successful food preservation represents more than just convenience. Our advanced methods of food preservation mean that much less food is lost to rodents, insects, and destructive microorganisms.

Antioxidants

Consider what happens to peaches, apples, and potatoes almost immediately after they are peeled. They quickly turn an unappealing brown color through a process called enzymatic browning, which results from a chemical reaction between oxygen in the air and enzymes in the food. Housewives have long known that dipping peeled vegetables and fruits into lemon, orange, or pineapple juice is a simple way to prevent them from browning. Most didn't realize, however, that this works because vitamin C in the juice is an antioxidant. (Antioxidants delay or prevent oxidation of foods, reactions in which oxygen combines with other substances and causes unpalatable flavors to develop.)

Food technologists have developed many other antioxidants to preserve a wide variety of foods. Antioxidants are especially important in preserving fatty foods like margarine, cooking oils, biscuits, salted nuts, and precooked dinners containing meat, fish, and poultry. Some antioxidants, such as citric acid, come from natural sources. Others, including BHT and BHA, are made by humans. Some antioxidants do double duty: they inhibit mold, yeast, and bacteria in addition to preventing oxidation.

Flavorants

"I can't eat it!" "It tastes terrible!" These cries are familiar to any parent who has tried to get a child to try a new food. The picky child makes a good point! No matter how healthful a food may be, it must taste good, or people simply won't eat it. Most people don't think of food as fuel for their biological machine but regard it as a source of pleasure. Flavorants, then, play an important role in ensuring that we all consume a nutritious diet.

Sir Raymond Priestly wrote an account of an expedition to Antarctica in 1910 in which a party that was marooned for nine months suffered severely from the harsh climate and the effects of starvation. Although eating raw seal blubber was their only option to prevent starvation, they couldn't choke it down until someone found a way to improve the terrible taste.

In a somewhat similar situation, scientists at the Institute of Nutrition of Central America in Panama were commissioned to develop an inexpensive, high-protein product for preventing the protein malnutrition that is so common in underdeveloped countries. They developed a very affordable complete protein from a combination of vegetable products (packaged and marketed under the name *Incaparina*). There was one major catch: the target population was repulsed by the product's taste, which was distinctly different from their culturally defined food preferences. Scientists finally modified this protein source to give it an acceptable corn flavor.

During the siege of Britain in World War II, as recounted by Dr. Melvin A. Benarde in *Our Precious Habitat,* Prime Minister Winston Churchill commanded his scientists to develop a nutrition plan that relied very little on food imports (at this difficult time, Britain depended heavily on food imports). Their recommendation: a diet of green vegetables, bread, and milk. Although this dietary plan was nutritionally complete, it was never adopted. The country's leaders feared that it was far too monotonous to gain acceptance. As British food scientist Magnus Pike commented:

> A diet may be perfectly balanced nutritionally, but if it is not sufficiently attractive, a workman may not eat enough of it to do his work. If a chemist can enhance the attractiveness of such a diet harmlessly, he is in fact contributing to nutritional well-being.

Without a doubt, then, we demand flavor in our food. Although there are many natural sources of flavor in our food supply, there just aren't enough to go around. For example, there isn't enough natural vanilla in the whole world to flavor the ice cream Americans eat in one year. To fill this gap, food technologists synthesize substances in the laboratory that have exactly the same taste as their "natural" counterparts. The laboratory-synthesized flavorants (often called "artificial") have the wonderful advantage of being available in virtually unlimited quantities. It's actually wrong to call these flavors "artificial" since they are identical in chemical structure to those found in nature. Just because they happen to be made in a laboratory doesn't make them unnatural. In fact, under German food law they are called "nature-identical."

Flavorants make up the largest single category of food additives. The FDA lists approximately twenty-eight hundred direct additives, the vast majority of which are flavors and spices. In addition to substances used directly as flavors, there are "flavor enhancers" such as MSG (monosodium glutamate), which make a person's taste buds more sensitive to certain flavors.

Emulsifiers

Emulsifiers are added to foods like salad dressing and chocolate milk to ensure that all ingredients—some of which don't naturally mix well—stay uniformly mixed to yield the desired taste and constituency. Lecithin, which occurs naturally in corn and soybeans, is widely used in foods as an emulsifier.

It's interesting to see how many of the people who condemn all "chemical food additives," which, of course, includes lecithin, see nothing inconsistent in dosing themselves with lecithin supplements. Some faddists even consume BHA and BHT with the belief that these antioxidants can retard their aging (oxidizing) processes.

Other Functions of Additives

We owe more to the chemicals used as food additives than just color, taste, consistency, and freshness. The list of jobs that additives do for us is long indeed.

• Maturing and bleaching agents used in wheat flour improve baking results. Freshly milled flour doesn't make a stable and elastic dough because it contains yellow pigmented proteins. Traditionally, flour was aged for approximately four months, during which time the yellow pigments were oxidized, allowing the flour to yield the desirable elastic dough. But such aging meant lost time and increased storage costs, not to mention an increased risk of molds, insects, and rodents invading the flour. Early in the nineteenth century, chemicals were discovered to speed up the maturing and bleaching processes. This treatment removes nothing from the flour and leaves no residue. It's just a matter of efficiency.

• Stabilizers and thickeners (including pectins, vegetable gums, and gelatins) give foods, such as ice cream, their uniform texture and desired consistency. A product with the consistency of slightly thickened milk—which is ice cream without stabilizers—could hardly be served in an ice-cream cone.

• Acids and bases control acidity and alkalinity in processed foods. These are added to cheese spreads and processed foods, for example, to obtain the desired texture and degree of tartness.

• Fortification of food with vitamins C and D and iodide has all but eliminated scurvy, rickets, and goiter. It just isn't accurate to describe enriched white bread as having been "stripped" of its natural goodness.

• Humectants help foods like coconut and marshmallows retain moisture.

• Anticaking agents keep powders and salts free-flowing.

• Curing agents, including salt, are used to cure and preserve meat.

• Foaming agents/foam inhibitors control the amount of air in food products.

• Leavening agents give foods a light texture.

This section provides only a brief overview of the role additives play in protecting and improving our food. For more detailed information on this subject, write for reprints to the *FDA Consumer,* Food and Drug Administration, 5600 Fishers Lane, Rockville, MD 20857 or to the Manufacturing Chemists Association, Inc, 1825 Connecticut Avenue N.W., Washington, DC 20009.

"Processing" Isn't a Four-Letter Word

For many consumers, the term "processed food" has taken on a negative meaning. "Health food" promoters like to describe processed foods as "natural foods that have been adulterated in some way to deceive the consumer and make extra money for the manufacturer."

Is this an accurate description? Exactly what is processing, anyway?

In the broadest sense, any product that is treated in any way once it leaves the farm is processed. Pasteurization of milk, for example, is a type of processing. It's difficult to understand why food faddists attack the pasteurization of milk, since this treatment kills microorganisms that cause milk to spoil. It also kills germs, such as salmonella, which can cause severe diarrhea and other serious symptoms. Pasteurization is so important that the

FDA has banned interstate sales of raw milk. Raw milk is still available for sale in some states where it is produced. In 1989 a California Superior Court judge ruled that the nation's largest raw milk producer, Alta-Dena Certified Dairy, and its affiliate, Steuve's Natural, had to stop advertising that raw milk is safer than pasteurized milk. The judge also ordered labels for raw milk informing consumers of the potential danger of bacterial infection associated with drinking unpasteurized milk and that the risks associated with bacterial contamination far outweigh any alleged health benefits.

Cheese processing is another target of many food faddists. Processed is made by combining a variety of cheeses (to ensure uniform flavor), heating them to the temperature necessary for pasteurization, and then pouring them into molds to cool. Since natural cheese separates into its component parts when heated, an emulsifier, usually a type of phosphate (not more than 3 percent phosphate by law), is added to keep the mixture homogenized. Sometimes cheese processors add salt (if it's lacking in the natural cheese base), and they are allowed to add up to 1 percent water to achieve the desired consistency.

Health faddists are also troubled by the addition of phosphate to cheese. They fail to recognize that phosphorus, in the form of phosphates and various organic compounds, is a necessary part of every cell and fluid in the body. The average daily adult intake of phosphorus in the United States is 1,500 to 1,600 mg, 20 to 30 percent of which may be provided by food additives. Processed cheese is not only wholesome and nutritious, but it offers certain advantages over raw cheese. It has a uniform taste and texture, doesn't dry out or mold as easily as other cheese, and doesn't always require refrigeration.

Using additives gives us the privilege of choosing from a wide variety of foods. Compare the selection available at your local supermarket to the foods on display at your local health food store. No wonder that even dedicated faddists may choose to "supplement" their diet with products from the mainstream food supply that are processed and contain additives.

The Nitrate/Nitrite Dilemma— Preventing a Deadly Disease

Botulism is a rare foodborne disease with a high fatality rate that develops after eating food contaminated by certain spore-forming bacteria. Symptoms of the disease, which usually strike between twelve and thirty-six hours after the tainted food is eaten, begin with nausea, vomiting, and paralysis of selected muscles and progress into double vision, drooping eyelids, dilated eyes, and often death.

The bacteria that cause botulism aren't killed by heating to the boiling point of water. A higher temperature is necessary to eliminate the deadly spores. People canning food at home should be careful to follow correct procedures, especially when canning nonacidic foods such as mushrooms.

Smoked meats offer another excellent breeding ground for botulism-causing bacteria. The best method of protecting these meat products is to use nitrates and nitrites. Although nitrates occur naturally in a number of vegetables, they are considered additives when used to cure meat. As was mentioned in the last chapter, it isn't nitrate itself that causes concern, but rather the conversion of nitrate to nitrite, which can then combine with common organic substances to form nitrosamines—a known carcinogen.

To protect human health with a generous margin of safety, the FDA has lowered the permissible levels of nitrate in foods. Allowed levels vary with the specific meat product: for example, cured meats such as bologna and salami, which aren't usually heated, are permitted to have higher levels than bacon, in which the cooking process can convert nitrates to nitrites. As an added safety measure, manufacturers add vitamin C to nitrate-containing products. Vitamin C blocks the formation of nitrosamines.

But let's put the whole issue of nitrates and nitrites into proper perspective. Their use greatly reduces our chance of falling victim to botulism—a risk with *proven* serious consequences. Cigarette smoking exposes smokers to up to ten times as many nitrosamines as food, water, and other sources in the environment combined!

Additives vs. Drugs

People who fear additives—who have nightmares of a white-coated scientist pouring the mysterious contents of a test tube into their chicken soup—may not think twice about taking prescription drugs. They simply accept the side effects that may accompany medication use.

Consider oral contraceptives, for example, which contain synthetic forms of estrogen and/or progesterone. Although questions have been raised, oral contraceptives are generally regarded as safe for women who are healthy and do not smoke cigarettes. These medications have been available for more than thirty years, and millions of women have chosen to take them. Yet our society has banned the use of DES (a synthetic estrogen) in cattle because it can result in insignificant traces of estrogen in beef liver (see Chapter 8).

The benefits of food additives may not be as apparent as those of drugs—not only for the consumer, but also for the health professional. But these very real benefits are sometimes even more dramatic than those of a "wonder drug."

But Are Additives Safe?

As you stew over the safety of chemicals added to food, remember:

• All foods are made up of chemicals. Just because the label on a milk carton reads "contains lactose, casein, lactalbumin, calcium, phosphorus," and more than one hundred other chemicals, don't feel that you need to serve it in a test tube.

• Food additives, especially those introduced in the last twenty-five years, have survived rigorous testing procedures. For example, before a food additive can be used, it must endure years of testing. All additives must be tested for acute, short-term, and long-term toxicity. Acute toxicity tests reveal what, if any, immediate effect a chemical has on a variety of laboratory animals. In short-term toxicity tests, (usually lasting about ninety days), varying amounts of the chemical are fed to animals. The animals are monitored for changes in general appearance, behavior, growth pattern, and, at autopsy, abnormalities in internal tissues and organs. Finally, long-term toxicity studies look for effects on fertility, reproduction, and the occurrence of cancer. Only additives that survive all three rounds of testing can gain FDA approval. These extensive procedures cost upwards of $100,000.

A petition for FDA approval includes all testing information, foods of intended use, amounts to be used in food, and labeling directions. An additive doesn't have a chance if it poses even the slightest threat to human health. The testing process is so rigorous that many "natural" substances—including vitamin A—could not survive it.

• Additives (not including common additives such as sugar and salt) make up less than 1 percent of the food we eat each year, and that includes spices and nutrients used in fortification. In light of this, it seems logical to worry less about additives and more about the safety of the other 99 percent. Of course, if an additive or food were shown to be hazardous to human health, then even "a little bit" might be too much to accept in our food supply. But constant food monitoring has found no such hazard or any evidence that various food chemicals are "stored up" to cause trouble later on.

• Allowed levels of food additives leave a generous margin of safety to protect human health. Strict regulations set allowed amounts at just one-hundredth of the level at which no adverse effects were shown in animals. This is a hundredfold margin of safety. As a matter of fact, the laws are so strict (as we'll see in later chapters) that some products have been removed from supermarket shelves before being given a full and fair trial. The FDA's policy is: guilty until proven innocent.

• There is no evidence linking food additives to any form of human disease or illness. The only type of cancer that has shown a dramatic increase since the 1940s, when additives began growing in popularity, is lung cancer. And there is no link between additives and lung cancer. In addition, heart disease, still our biggest killer, hasn't been linked to the use of additives.

• Consumers are in far greater danger from improper food preparation and storage than from food additives. Both of these problem areas pale in comparison to the adverse health effects of overeating.

In the next chapter, we'll touch briefly on the history of food safety legislation and then examine the pros and cons of the famous (or infamous) Delaney anticancer clause.

7

The Delaney Dilemma

"For instance, now. . . there's the King's
   Messenger.
He's in prison now, being punished; and
   the trial doesn't even begin till next
   Wednesday and, of course, the crime
   comes last of all."

—Lewis Carroll
Through the Looking Glass

Food Regulation—The Beginnings

As nearly as we can tell, the first English food law, known as the
Assize of Bread, was enacted by King John in 1202. It strictly
prohibited the substitution of peas or beans for flour in bread.

The first general food law in the United States was created
in 1784 when Massachusetts enacted "an act against selling
unwholesome provisions." Food regulation activity picked up
in the nineteenth century with the passage of several state and
federal acts calling for the inspection of food, tea, and other
beverages, and of animals before slaughter.

Today's complex food regulations began to develop around
the turn of this century. These regulations came in response to

125

urbanization: as people moved from the country to the city, they became more dependent on purchased foodstuffs. Seizing the opportunity, "get-rich-quick" seekers sold food products that were less-than-wholesome—even adulterated and unsafe—for a fat profit. Upton Sinclair's 1906 book, *The Jungle,* vividly reported the filthy conditions under which meat and meat products were processed in Chicago. The public was horrified and outraged. As Sinclair put it, "I aimed at the public's heart and by accident I hit it in the stomach."

Another important figure in the history of food safety was chemist Dr. Harvey Washington Wiley of the United States Department of Agriculture (USDA). He personally accepted responsibility for monitoring the United States food supply. Wiley formed what became known as the "Wiley poison squad": twelve healthy young men who became human guinea pigs by pledging to eat nothing but the food Dr. Wiley gave them. If any of them showed any sign of illness after eating test food, that food was labeled "suspect." In fact, it would be seriously considered for removal from the marketplace.

Today, instead of a "poison squad," the FDA uses laboratory animals and force-feeds them amounts of different substances that are many times the equivalent of normal human consumption. Test animals are then dissected and scrutinized for signs of tumors and other abnormalities.

Wiley and his brave (or perhaps foolhardy) associates set the stage for modern food legislation. Recommendations based on the poison squad's findings prompted passage of the Pure Food and Drug Act of 1906, which was also called the "Wiley Act." This law required that chemicals added to foods pass a test showing that they are safe and serve a useful purpose. The act condemned "any added poisonous or other added deleterious ingredients which may render such article injurious to health." The Food, Drug, and Insecticide Administration—formed in

1927 to enforce food, drug, and cosmetic legislation—was renamed the Food and Drug Administration in 1931.

Loopholes in the 1906 legislation became apparent. One loophole even allowed the marketing of an untested elixir of sulfanilamide, a sulfa drug that contained a solvent that killed 107 people, mostly children. Largely in response to the Elixir of Sulfanilamide tragedy, Congress passed the 1938 Food, Drug, and Cosmetic Act in an effort to prevent foods and drugs from being marketed before they had been cleared for safety.

This act raised interesting issues. Would manufacturers, for example, have to prove the safety of food additives already in use for many years? What about salt and sugar—would they have to undergo extensive testing? In 1958 Congress enacted the Food Additives Amendment to the Food, Drug, and Cosmetic Act. This legislation required that substances intentionally added to food, or entering the food during processing, storage, or packaging, be cleared for safety before marketing. In response, the FDA divided food additives into four categories:

1. *"Prior sanctioned" substances*. Substances that had previously received official approval for special purposes were granted "grandfather" status.

2. Substances *"generally recognized as safe."* The well-known GRAS list originally included almost seven hundred substances, including ascorbic acid (vitamin C), caffeine, cinnamon, MSG, BHA, BHT, sugar, pepper, mustard seed, cyclamates, and saccharin, all of which had been approved by the FDA based on published scientific testing or a history of safe use.

3. *Food Colors*. Dyes used in foods, drugs, cosmetics, and medical devices had to undergo premarket testing similar to that for food additives.

4. *Food additives*. Substances that had not been proved safe had to undergo rigorous testing before being allowed in the food supply.

Although this legislation excluded prior-sanctioned and GRAS substances from the definition of "food additives," the term additive is used in its more general sense throughout this book.

Forty-Seven Words

It wasn't until 1958 that manufacturers were required to prove that additives to food products were safe *before* they hit the market. At first glance, the 1958 law seemed to provide an ideal balance between legislative control and scientific judgment. But in the final hours of debate, Congress voted to add forty-seven carefully chosen words that significantly changed the impact of the amendment. The so-called Delaney Clause banned from the food supply any additive that caused cancer in humans *or animals* with the words:

> No additive shall be deemed to be safe if it is found to induce cancer when ingested by man or animal or if it is found, after tests which are appropriate for the evaluation of the safety of food additives, to induce cancer in man or animals.

In retrospect, the Delaney Clause was a knee-jerk response to an increasing cancer death rate. Then, as today, cancer was the third leading cause of death and a focus of fear and misunderstanding. Proponents of the Delaney Clause clamored for drastic measures to reduce the rate of this mysterious scourge by targeting food additives. When asked why cancer was used to ascertain additive safety, Mr. Delaney replied: "Cancer is the most horrible of all diseases. . . . What else would you single out?"

Invoking the Delaney Clause can be likened to plowing your rose bed to rid it of weeds. You'll get rid of the weeds, but you'll also get rid of your roses. Today we are stuck with a law that can ban a substance without regard to the size of the dose used in testing or the species tested. No ifs, ands, or buts. Or rational thinking. In fact, some experts believe that this "anticancer" clause may have been a primary impetus for today's panic-in-the-pantry phenomenon.

The Delaney Clause was originally applied to additives for which approval was requested and not to additives deemed "previously sanctioned" or on the GRAS list. Later, the clause's reach was extended to cover color additives (1960) and residues of animal drugs in meat, eggs, and milk (1968). Of course, if a previously approved additive could be shown to cause cancer, the Delaney Clause could be invoked to ban it. But let's backtrack for a moment and discuss the intended advantages of the Delaney Clause.

In Defense of Delaney

Dr. G. Burroughs Midler, associate director of the National Cancer Institute in 1958, believed that the Delaney Clause was the missing artillery in the war against cancer. In line with his belief, he said: "No one at this time can tell how much or how little of a carcinogen will be required to produce cancer in any human being, or how long it would take the cancer to develop." He argued that any chemical linked to cancer—even remotely so—should be banned. He and others believed that there was always the danger that carcinogens accumulated in the body. Such chemicals, they feared, could combine to pose a significant problem that neither posed by itself.

In 1973, the spirit of the Delaney Clause was supported by the New York Academy of Sciences, which recommended avoiding exposure to food additives shown to be even mildly carcinogenic in animals. These scientists went even further than Delaney, recommending that efforts be extended to avoid such questionable chemicals in air and water.

Attorney James S. Turner, author of *The Chemical Feast,* expressed his agreement with the Delaney Clause in the *Vanderbilt Law Review.* He called the Delaney Clause a "model environmental protection law," and, like the New York Academy of Sciences, felt it should have more far-reaching applications. Turner was especially impressed with the clause's provision for appropriating responsibility to both scientists and to Congress: scientists were charged with making responsible scientific judgments on the basis of test results, and Congress with making sound policy decisions. Unfortunately, this process has never worked.

Delaney's Beliefs

Representative James J. Delaney, the dominant figure behind the passage of this controversial anticancer clause recalled: "We worked the language back and forth, back and forth . . . on such a small clause as that we dotted every i and crossed every t . . . until we had something we thought could be understood by the public." He explained that use of the word ingest, for example, which commonly means to take food, drink, or other substances into the stomach by swallowing, wasn't accidental, but was the result of careful thought.

What drove Mr. Delaney?

First of all, he was suspicious of technology's supposed ability to improve on nature. He recalled his childhood when he would take a spoonful of Baker's chocolate and put it in hot water with some sugar, only to find that the two substances wouldn't mix. But today's products, he pointed out, contain emulsifiers that are "so powerful (they) can tear down these molecules and make oil mix with water." Although admitting that this mixing process was a "great improvement from a commercial standpoint," he naively expressed concern about its possible effects on the body, the liver, and the spleen. His conclusion that "such chemicals must build up residual toxicity in the body" sparked his interest in the "problem."

Secondly, Delaney was suspicious of the FDA. He said, "There's nobody, so to speak, on my side except some dedicated professor emeritus. Food and Drug is supposed to protect the health of the public. . . . you wonder what side they are on. They're with the manufacturers as far as I can see." Delaney also said that "carcinogens are subtle, stealthy, sinister saboteurs of life. They have no place in our food chain. . . . Chemicals do not have rights. People do."

Undoubtedly, Delaney was sincere. But sincerity in belief is not the same as belief rooted in scientific fact. The Delaney Clause mixed politics with scientific fact, something that even the best emulsifiers do not accomplish smoothly.

More Questions Than Answers

The Delaney Clause wasn't the answer to the cancer question. Indeed, its inflexibility and inconsistency are illustrated by the following points:

• *The wording of the Delaney Clause leaves little if any room for scientific judgment.* The forty-seven words called for a total ban of any substance shown to cause cancer in humans or animals, regardless of dose or testing protocol. The atmosphere of fear and urgency created by the arbitrary nature of the clause has contributed to public concern about food safety to a degree not supported by true, unbiased scientific inquiry.

History has proved this point several times. The Delaney red flag is desperately waved, in fact, even when cancer is simply *suspected* (as we illustrate with artificial sweeteners in chapter 8). Because of the Delaney Clause, food regulation has become a matter of political evaluation of scientific information, not in-depth scientific reasoning.

• *There is no give-and-take in the Delaney Clause—no room for analysis of benefit versus risk.* Consider the case of DDT, a chemical which has saved more lives and prevented more disease than any other chemical in history. DDT was especially valuable in reducing morbidity and mortality from malaria. In Ceylon (now Sri Lanka), for example, the number of deaths exceeded two million per year before DDT was used. With DDT spraying, the number was reduced to a mere seventeen per year. But because of studies in which DDT-eating mice developed tumors, DDT was banned. Five years later, malarial deaths in Sri Lanka again exceeded two million.

• *It isn't consistent to use the Delaney Clause to ban all food additives that have been implicated in causing cancer in animals while ignoring the fact that many natural foods not only contribute to the development of cancer, but are also considered more harmful (even lethal) in other ways.* As we read in chapter 4, "natural" isn't always without risk and is definitely not cancer-free! Nonetheless, the Delaney Clause basically grants immunity to natural substances while putting additives through the mill.

• *There's the question of how accurately cancer tests in animals predict human cancer risk.* Consider for example, the widely publicized experiment in which rats were fed saccharin at a level equivalent to a human daily dose of eight hundred cans of saccharin-containing diet soft drink. The bladder tumors found in the rats led to an attempt to ban the sweetener. Recent research suggests that the high doses of saccharin may cause bladder cancer only in rats and not in mice, other animals, or humans. Another new explanation, offered by Dr. Bruce Ames, is that high dosage, not the nature of the substance, is what triggers development of the cancer.

Sound science dictates that higher-than-normal human doses of additives be used in animal tests so that these tests can detect cancer risk in a relatively short period of time. However, evaluations of such tests should be based on rational scientific thinking. The public should question the power of the Delaney Clause to automatically ban a substance on the basis of *any* experiment testing *any* substance at *any* dose and for *any* length of time. To be sure, common sense suggests that too much of anything can harm people. Too much sun, for example, can cause skin cancer. But that certainly doesn't mean that people should stay indoors 100 percent of the time.

• *It's a well known fact that there are significant differences in an animal's susceptibility to develop cancer, yet the Delaney Clause doesn't allow for this interspecies difference.* One strain of rats exposed to chemical A may not develop cancer as a result of that exposure. One hundred percent of another rat strain, however, may develop cancer after identical exposure to chemical A. Dr. Elizabeth Weisburger, formerly of the National Cancer Institute, pointed out that increased cancer susceptibility can even be caused by a bladder parasite. This inter- and intraspecies difference in cancer susceptibility has two implications for the Delaney Clause: (1) the risk of cancer from a substance may be overestimated because test animals may have some susceptibility-increasing factor (like the bladder parasite), and (2) the risk of cancer may be underestimated because a particularly hardy strain or species was chosen for the test.

Animal-to-human extrapolation presents several other problems. Drs. D. Mark Hegsted and Lynne Ausman of Harvard's

Department of Nutrition have identified three differences between humans and animals: (1) distinct metabolic pathways (or ways of digesting, using, and storing substances within the body), (2) varying nutritional requirements (baby rats, for example, grow so rapidly that it is improper to compare their nutritional needs to those of a human baby), and (3) differences in the ability to detoxify foreign substances that enter the body.

• *Dr. Weisburger also notes that "as [scientific] methods become more sensitive, [scientists] can find compounds where it was thought there were no traces of these [foreign] materials."* In other words, what is the significance of what scientists are detecting? If cancer is detected, for example, after exposure to an extremely low concentration of a chemical (a level only measurable because of exquisitely sensitive testing equipment), can scientists be certain that the presence of the chemical and the development of cancer are truly related?

Today's equipment, which can measure some substances in picogram amounts (trillionths of a gram), is sensitive enough to find a trace of just about anything in anything. (This is illustrated in the next chapter by the cattle-growth stimulant DES.) This drawback of the Delaney Clause has become even more of a problem as screening techniques have continued to increase in sophistication.

• *People puzzled by the Delaney Clause ask, "Why is it limited to cancer? What about other diseases that might be linked to food?"* Questions like these have to be asked very carefully to prevent the potential disaster of *expanding* the Delaney Clause. Senator Gaylord Nelson wanted to broaden the Delaney Clause to state that no food additive would be acceptable if it induced any biological injury or damage of any type, including, but not limited to, the induction of cancer, birth defects, and mutational changes.

Dr. Julius M. Coon, professor of pharmacology at Thomas Jefferson University, explained the potential problems of this approach:

> If such a bill became law, it would create utter chaos in toxicologic circles and in government regulatory agencies as well. It would be a real challenge, if not impossible, to find any additive that would not cause some harmful effects in test animals fed high levels over a long period of time. Strict interpretation of this law, for example, would quickly disqualify salt, sugar, vitamins A and D, and iron salts as food additives.

These problems with the strict application of the Delaney Clause are illustrated in the next chapter by three examples that have had widespread effects on the American public: DES, artificial sweeteners, and Red Dye No. 3.

8

(Mis)Applying Delaney

"Were you ever punished?"
"Only for faults," said Alice.
"And you were all the better for it, I
know!" the Queen said triumphantly.
"Yes, but then I had done the things I was
punished for," said Alice.
"That makes all the difference.'"

—Lewis Carroll
Through the Looking Glass

The Beef Over DES

DES (short for the tongue-twisting diethylstilbestrol) is a synthetic form of estrogen. It's been available since the 1940s as a medication and in 1973 was approved for emergency use as a "morning-after" contraceptive pill.

DES was used as a growth stimulant in cattle from 1954 through 1972. When properly used with a steer, it can stimulate a five-hundred-pound animal to reach a marketable weight of one thousand pounds in thirty-four days less time *and* with five hundred pounds less feed than an animal not receiving DES.

137

DES also has desirable effects on meat quality: it increases protein and moisture by 7 percent, thereby decreasing the percentage of fat in that meat. Prior to its 1972 banning, DES was fed to 75 percent of the thirty million cattle slaughtered each year in the United States.

When DES use in cattle began, it did not have a clear safety record. Experts had known since 1940 that DES, like all types of estrogen, causes cancer in test animals—breast cancer in mice and rats and testicular cancer in mice. When the Delaney Clause was adopted in 1958, cattle industry experts, together with government officials, searched the fine print of Delaney to allow the continued use of DES. They concluded that DES could be used as long as no residue was found in the meat.

In 1959, though, residues were found in chickens, resulting in the immediate banning of DES use in poultry. But its use in beef remained legal as long as no residue could be found. As a precautionary measure, cattle farmers were required to stop using DES in their animals forty-eight hours before slaughter.

Cattle farmers continued to use DES in beef cattle during the 1960s. The testing methods had improved, allowing the detection of levels as minute as ten parts per billion of a substance in another substance (which is about the same as five drops per twenty-five thousand gallons of water). DES was still immune from Delaney's grasp because either it wasn't found at all in beef, or was at levels below the ability to detect it.

Rare Vaginal Cancer Causes Alarm

In 1971 Dr. Arthur Herbst, a gynecologist at Massachusetts General Hospital, reported a link between young women with an extremely rare form of vaginal cancer (adenocarcinoma) and their mothers' use of DES during pregnancy. (DES was used to decrease the risk of miscarriage.) Publication of his findings in the *New England Journal of Medicine* raised a red flag about the safety of DES use in cattle. By the end of 1971 the pressure was on and DES use in animals was severely criticized. Cattle raisers were told to withdraw the drug seven days before slaughter, and residue testing continued.

By 1972 a highly sensitive form of radioactive tracer technique became available, and DES residues were found in the livers of about 2.5 percent of randomly selected animals. In July 1972 Senator Edward Kennedy held a subcommittee hearing and further alarmed the public with the words: "We are here today because DES, a known cancer-causing agent, is appearing on thousands of American dinner tables."

Americans were up in arms. They didn't want any cancer-causing hormones in their hamburgers. An "us-versus-them" attitude was orchestrated by critics who described DES as a means of "saving cattlemen some $90 million yearly." Of course, they didn't stop to think that it wasn't just cattlemen who were saving money, but the public that benefited through lower-priced beef products.

Inconsistencies in the Banning of DES

In their concern over their meatloaf, consumers failed to seek out essential facts.

• DES is not the only source of estrogen in the food supply. Milk, eggs, and even honey contain estrogen. It's been estimated that one egg provides one thousand times the amount of estrogen found in a serving of liver from a DES-treated animal. Birth control pills, which many women use almost daily, contain far more synthetic estrogen than does a serving of liver containing DES.

• Even more basic, a woman's body regularly produces estrogens. (Men also produce some, but not as much as women.) The prestigious British science journal *Nature* estimated that it would take five hundred pounds of liver containing two parts per billion of DES to equal the amount of estrogen produced each day by a woman during her reproductive years.

• Women who were treated with estrogen to prevent miscarriage received up to 125 mg a day during pregnancy. To get that same amount of estrogen, a woman would have to eat 62.5 tons of beef liver (containing two parts per billion of DES) at one sitting. And the amount of estrogen used in the DES "morning-after" birth-control method would be equivalent to eating a 500-ton serving of liver containing DES residues.

• DES was condemned in spite of the fact that there was no evidence that the tiny traces of DES in beef liver were harmful to humans or animals.

• All evidence points to the fact that there is a "no-effect" level for DES and other estrogens. The no-effect level is that level of a substance that doesn't cause tumors or other health problems. This "no-effect" principle has been demonstrated in mice. All of us, male and female, have natural levels of estrogen. The fact that most people don't develop cancer suggests that the same principle holds true for humans.

It was indeed alarming to find out that massive doses of DES given to women during pregnancy could contribute to the development of cancer in some of their daughters. As alarming as it was, however, this observation shouldn't have been applied to the inconsequential traces of estrogen in food, *especially* in light of our own natural estrogen production.

But hysteria and politics teamed up. In August 1972, FDA Commissioner Charles C. Edwards announced that he had "no choice" but to discontinue approval for DES in animal feed. His ruling still allowed slow-release DES implants in animals' ears. But less than a year later, the FDA banned these implants after 0.04 to 0.12 parts per billion of DES were found in beef liver from animals treated with them.

In protest, the manufacturers of DES requested an FDA hearing. When the FDA refused, the manufacturers appealed. In January 1974, the United States Court of Appeals ruled that the FDA's orders were invalid and that the manufacturers of DES could resume marketing their products until the agency had held a hearing. The court took action because:

> The FDA chose to act summarily, without a hearing, without making known to petitioners the nature of the "new evidence" or of the underlying tests, and without giving the petitioners an opportunity to controvert the new evidence.

In the end, the FDA prevailed. In 1979, the manufacturers and cattle farmers lost a hard-fought court fight and DES was banned from livestock use.

The struggle over DES is only one example of the effect the Delaney Clause has had on our food supply. Perhaps the best known debate over the Delaney Clause has been in the area of artificial sweeteners.

The American Sweet Tooth

Although some food faddists would have you believe that your sweet tooth is the result of habits you formed as a child, research has proved that infants are *born* with a preference for a sweet taste. Our ancient ancestors used fruits and the sweet parts of plants to satisfy their liking for sweets. As early as 2500 B.C., the Egyptians kept bees for the honey they could produce. The ancient Romans and Greeks pressed sugar cane for its sweet juice. And by the tenth century, the Egyptians used chemical methods to refine sugar.

Americans are known the world over for their demanding sweet tooth. Food and beverage manufacturers gladly respond with an ample supply of products to satisfy this never-ending hunger for sweets. Before delving into the history of non-nutritive (artificial) sweeteners, let's look at some facts about nutritive (calorie-containing) sweeteners:

• Sucrose (table sugar) occurs naturally in fruits and is added to many foods.

• Fructose, which is up to 1.5 times as sweet as sucrose, occurs naturally in fruit and is used in some food products.

• Lactose, or milk sugar, occurs naturally in milk and dairy products. It is added to many food items—not to impart sweetness, since it is only 10 percent as sweet as sucrose—but as a filler or bulking agent.

• Corn syrup is often used instead of sucrose in foods because it is less sweet than sugar and also provides texture

• High-fructose corn syrup (HFCS), consisting of 40 to 100 percent fructose, is sweeter than sucrose and allows for slightly lower-calorie products.

• Sugar alcohols—such as sorbitol, mannitol, maltitol, and xylitol—occur naturally in fruits and are often used in reduced-calorie foods, as well as in foods for diabetics.

• All of these sweeteners except xylitol are less sweet than sucrose.

• Aspartame, which is formed from two amino acids, phenylalanine and methyl aspartate, is about 180 times sweeter than sugar and can be used in much smaller quantities. It is considered a nutritive sweetener because it provides the same calories as protein.

In 1976 Americans purchased an average of 93.4 pounds of sucrose and 7.2 pounds of HFCS, for a total of 124.4 pounds of nutritive sweeteners—and consumed approximately 75-80 percent of this quantity. Americans in 1986 consumed almost the same total amount of nutritive sweeteners, but were consuming less sucrose and much more high-fructose corn syrup (which probably represents increased consumption of more pre-sweetened items).

The Sugar Scare

At various times, sugar has been accused of causing diabetes, hypoglycemia, coronary heart disease, obesity, and tooth decay. Let's take a look at these claims and the relevant facts.

• Even in excess amounts, sugar does not *cause* diabetes. Consuming large amounts of sugar, however, may make this disease worse.

• For many years, hypoglycemia was "in." Many people experiencing tiredness, headaches, and weakness were relieved to finally have identified a cause for their everyday symptoms. In some people the pancreas produces too much insulin in response to the normal elevation of blood sugar levels after eating; but this abnormality is rare. Contrary to popular opinion, sucrose and other concentrated sweets do not cause hypoglycemia.

• A few years ago Dr. John Yudkin, a British physician, suggested that sucrose might play a role in causing coronary heart disease (CHD). His theory was widely circulated by faddists, but mainstream scientists have never thought it was correct.

• Obesity, which plagues nearly 40 percent of Americans, occurs when a person consumes more calories than are burned up. Sugar, starch, protein, fat, and alcohol all provide calories—and sugar alone is seldom the real culprit. Fat provides more calories per gram than sugar (and starch, protein, and alcohol), and excess fat intake is more often to blame for than excess sugar intake. In fact, recent evidence suggests that high-fat diets are more likely than high-carbohydrate diets to produce obesity.

Sugar, then, has been cleared of all charges except of contributing to tooth decay, especially when it is in a sticky form and is consumed in large quantities between meals. Facts withstanding, antisugar activists continue their campaign against sugar, saying that it shouldn't even be considered a nutrient.

Sugar *is* a legitimate nutrient. It is simple, digestible, pure carbohydrate. Perhaps the feeling that sugar shouldn't be a nutrient stems from the practice of using the word nutrient in a more limited sense to indicate *essential* nutrient. Actually, sugar and other carbohydrates are nutrients and important sources of relatively inexpensive energy. Beyond its contributions to flavor and energy, sugar also can function as a preservative and as a jellying and fermenting agent.

The Ups and Downs of Artificial Sweeteners

More than a century ago, scientists began searching for calorie-free artificial sweeteners to replace sugar and other nutritive sweeteners in the diet of diabetics. While this relatively small segment of the population enjoyed such products, other people indulged their sweet tooth with the real thing.

But then the 1960s hit, bringing with them an increasing focus on healthy lifestyle. Overweight was shunned as a risk to good health and long life. Physical attractiveness was defined by ever-slimmer fashion models, and the urge to purge those extra pounds became ever stronger. Nondiabetics soon turned to artificial sweeteners in an effort to reduce calories, yet satisfy their sweet tooth. Sales of these noncaloric sweeteners grew tremendously, both as table sweeteners and as ingredients in a variety of foods.

Cyclamate, discovered in 1937, is about thirty times sweeter than sugar, is chemically stable, leaves no aftertaste, and is inexpensive to produce. It was originally approved for use in products for diabetic and obese patients in 1951 but was reclassified for general use after the passage of the 1958 food additive legislation.

Sweet dreams soon turned to nightmares! In 1968 doubts were raised about cyclamate's safety, and a 1969 study linked the sweetener to the development of cancer in laboratory rats. The Delaney Clause was invoked, and cyclamate lost its place on the FDA's "generally recognized as safe" (GRAS) list. At the time cyclamate was removed from the U.S. food supply, market analysts estimated that as much as 75 percent of the population used some form of this sweetener. Product recalls were very costly to the food industry.

Cyclamate's manufacturer, Abbott Laboratories, has tried repeatedly to get its product reestablished, arguing that the condemning research was seriously flawed and unreliable. Two years after a 1975 National Cancer Institute study concluded that "the present evidence does not establish the carcinogenicity of cyclamate," Abbott petitioned the FDA for a new ruling, but the FDA replied that Abbott hadn't proved with any certainty that cyclamate doesn't cause cancer. Abbott tried again in 1982 after the ban against cyclamate had been removed in many foreign countries. The following year the FDA asked the National Research Council (NRC) to conduct a review of all the evidence on cyclamate. The NRC's report, which took two years to prepare, concluded that cyclamate is not carcinogenic. In spite of overwhelming evidence that cyclamate is safe, the FDA still has not allowed cyclamate back into the American market.

Saccharin was discovered in 1879 and was the first sweetener marketed in the United States. Cheap to produce, saccharin is about three hundred times sweeter than sugar, has a long shelf life, and combines well with other sweeteners. Saccharin's only drawback for much of its career was its slightly bitter aftertaste.

From its introduction, saccharin was very popular, especially in Europe during World War II, when sugar was rationed. Sales of the artificial sweetener shot up dramatically when manufacturers introduced diet soft drinks sweetened with saccharin.

In the early 1960s both cyclamate and saccharin were available and were often combined. Food technologists discovered that a mixture of ten parts cyclamate to one part saccharin produced a stable product with the desired sweet taste and without any bitter aftertaste. Although consumers were still charged a higher price for a "special food product," many of these items, such as diet soft drinks, actually cost less to produce than those with sugar.

After cyclamate was removed from the market, manufacturers sometimes combined saccharin with sugar to combat its bitter aftertaste. Then, barely six months after the ban on cyclamate, more bad news hit the artificially sweetened food industry. A research study found that saccharin could cause bladder cancer in mice. Even though the FDA didn't act on the researcher's evidence, the seeds of doubt had been sown. When a second study (in 1972) showed a saccharin-cancer association, saccharin was removed from the GRAS list until further study could be done. After a 1977 Canadian study found that saccharin caused bladder cancer in rats, the FDA proposed a total ban.

But then something unusual happened. Diabetics pressured the FDA to remove the ban, since no other nonnutritive sweeteners were available at that time. Congress held hearings to review the FDA decision and finally imposed a moratorium on the ban—at least until the FDA could conduct its own research to evaluate saccharin's safety. Saccharin products were soon back on the market, but manufacturers were required to add a warning label. The moratorium was renewed in 1979 and has been extended several times. Its present deadline is in 1997. In 1991 the FDA withdrew its proposal to ban saccharin, stating that it was outdated. The warning label imposed by Congress, however, is still required.

Aspartame entered the market during all the hullabaloo over saccharin and cyclamates. Aspartame was accidentally discovered in 1965 by a research worker in a laboratory at G. D. Searle who observed that a compound made of two amino acids (phenylalanine and aspartic acid) and methyl alcohol tasted very sweet. Although this particular combination doesn't appear in nature, amino acids are the building blocks of protein, and small amounts of methyl alcohol occur naturally in some foods.

Aspartame has no aftertaste, but it isn't as stable as cyclamate, is much more expensive than saccharin, and can't be used in baking because it breaks down and loses its sweet taste when heated for a prolonged period. Aspartame also differs from both cyclamate and saccharin in that it does provide some calories when its three components are metabolized. However, since it is about 180 times sweeter than sugar, its caloric contribution to the diet is insignificant.

Considering the history of cyclamate and saccharin, it isn't surprising that aspartame has encountered controversy from its beginnings. The G.D. Searle Company spent years conducting research on aspartame before it received FDA approval for the product in 1974. Before it hit the market, however, new questions were raised about the safety of two of its breakdown products—phenylalanine and methyl alcohol—and the FDA suspended its approval.

Before these questions could be answered, a new controversy arose. Some researchers claimed that Searle had supplied inaccurate information to the FDA. Although these charges never were proved, the FDA and the Universities Associated for Research and Evaluation in Pathology investigated Searle's research data. In 1981, after a six-year delay, Searle's data were deemed accurate, and aspartame was finally approved for use as a table-top sweetener and in certain foods and beverages. By 1983 aspartame was allowed in soft drinks. Since that time, aspartame, which is marketed under the brand names *NutraSweet* (used in food products) and *Equal* (a tabletop sweetener), has become a billion-dollar business.

Unlike cyclamates and saccharin, aspartame has not been associated with cancer in laboratory animal tests. Beginning in the mid-1980s, however, the FDA and the U.S. Centers for Disease Control (CDC) investigated consumer complaints of nausea, diarrhea, headaches, mood changes, seizures, and anxiety, all of which were blamed on aspartame.

In 1985 both the CDC and the American Medical Association's Council on Scientific Affairs concluded that there was no evidence that aspartame represented a health risk to any group except people with phenylketonuria (PKU), a disease in which people cannot metabolize phenylalanine. Other scientists scrutinized aspartame and conducted a number of double-blind studies. Duke University researchers, for example, studied people who complained of headache after ingesting aspartame and found that these people were no more likely to have a headache when receiving the amount of aspartame in a gallon of diet soft drink than when they were given a placebo. At the National Institute of Mental Health, a similar study investigated claims that aspartame causes disruptive behavior in preschool children and failed to find such a link.

The FDA has set an "Acceptable Daily Intake" of fifty milligrams of aspartame for each kilogram (2.2 pounds) of body weight. This means that a 150-pound person would have to drink twenty cans of aspartame-sweetened soft drink per day to reach this suggested limit.

Acesulfame-K was invented by West German scientists of Hoechst Company in 1967. This compound, marketed as Sunette, is two hundred times sweeter than sugar and leaves no aftertaste. It passes through the body without being changed and, unlike aspartame, is not broken down by heat. In mid-1988 the FDA approved acesulfame-K for use in powdered drink mixes, puddings, chewing gum, and tabletop sweeteners. (The K stands for potassium.) Shortly before acesulfame-K was approved, the Center for Science in the Public Interest (CSPI) began a series of allegations that animal studies indicate risks of lung cancer, mammary tumors, and elevated cholesterol. Early in 1992, the FDA denied the group's request for a formal public hearing and stated that the studies conducted to test the new sweetener had been adequate to demonstrate its safety.

Alitame resulted from research conducted by Pfizer, Inc., to develop an artificial sweetener similar to aspartame. Alitame is composed of two amino acids, L-aspartic acid and D-alanine. It is considered a caloric sweetener because it provides almost 1.5 calories per gram. Because of its extreme sweetness (about 2,000 times as sweet as sugar), however, the amounts needed in food will be tiny. Alitame can be used in baking, but it is somewhat unstable in acidic solutions. Although extensive research has shown it to be safe, the FDA has not yet acted on the manufacturer's petition for approval as a food additive.

Sucralose, as its name suggests, is made from ordinary table sugar (sucrose), but it is 600 times sweeter. Sucralose is suitable for use in many food products. It does not break down in the body and provides no calories. Although CSPI (as usual) has questioned its safety, sucralose has been thoroughly investigated in Canada and has been accepted by the Joint FAO/WHO Expert Committee on Food Additives. Sucralose was approved for use in Canada in 1991, but the petition of McNeil Specialty Products Co. for approval as a food additive in the U.S. is still under consideration by the FDA.

Several other nonnutritive sweeteners are in various stages of research and development, waiting to cash in on the financially rewarding reduced-calorie segment of the food marketplace. *L-sugars,* for example, are mirror images of regular sugar molecules. Although their sweetness is similar to their regular counterparts, they are not broken down in the body and therefore provide no calories. *Stevioside* (also called *Stevia*) is a sweetener made from a South American plant and is already marketed in Japan and several other countries. It is about 300 times sweeter than table sugar. *Dihydrochalcone* sweeteners are derived from bitter flavonone compounds that are present in citrus fruits. Developers of these substances do not expect safety to become an issue because they are similar to the naturally occurring flavonoids found in everyday foods.

Interestingly, studies have failed to show a relationship between using noncaloric sweeteners and weight loss—the primary reason they have become so popular. Dieters apparently make up for the calories saved from using noncaloric sweeteners by eating more of other foods. A 1960s study from Harvard's Department of Nutrition followed more than three hundred obese individuals for three years. Approximately half of these subjects used either saccharin or cyclamate; half didn't use a noncaloric sweetener. There was no difference in weight gain or loss between the various groups during the three-year period.

An Issue Colored by Politics

FD&C Red No. 3 is the last of the food colors reviewed by the FDA. It was tested in the 1960s and was permanently listed for use in foods in 1969. In 1982 the International Research and Development Corporation conducted studies that showed that Red No. 3 causes thyroid cancer in male rats. This prompted an invocation of the Delaney Clause.

Early in 1990, the FDA banned the provisional uses of Red No. 3, which accounted for about one-fifth of all uses of the dye—in such items as lipsticks, pill coatings, baked goods, ice cream, cosmetics, and externally applied drugs. This action does not affect the permanently approved uses, such as in fruit juices, gelatin desserts, and fruit cocktail cherries. In announcing the ban on provisional uses, the FDA reassured consumers that the risk associated with using such items is so small as to be negligible. In fact, consumers were encouraged to use up existing supplies of products containing Red No. 3. In a January 29, 1990 press release, the FDA said:

> Under the so-called Delaney Clause of the 1960 Color Additive amendments to the Food, Drug and Cosmetics Act, products shown to have carcinogenic effect in laboratory tests, no matter how small, cannot be approved for use by FDA. The decision to ban the uses of Red No. 3, therefore, is not based on risk but on the legal mandate of the Delaney Clause.

The scientifically unnecessary but politically motivated partial ban on Red No. 3 forced the FDA to take a critical look at food safety regulation. The January 29 press release also noted:

> The National Academy of Sciences has recommended that the Delaney Clause be replaced by a "negligible risk" standard, especially to reflect significant technological advances since 1960 in the detection of low levels of carcinogenic substances. The Administration is concerned about the rigidity of the Delaney Clause and has proposed a change on a similar risk assessment issue involving pesticides in foods as part of its food safety initiative announced last fall.

Legislation has been introduced that would substitute a "negligible-risk" standard for the "zero-risk" standard in the Delaney Clause. Such legislation was endorsed by President Bush in his October 1989 Food Safety Plan. It remains to be seen whether a law of this type will be enacted.

9

Fears and Foibles:
The Aftershock of Delaney

"Let the jury consider their verdict," the
King said, for about the twentieth
time that day.
"No, no!" said the Queen. "Sentence
first, verdict afterwards."
"Stuff and nonsense!" said Alice loudly.
"The idea of having the sentence first!"

—Lewis Carroll
Alice in Wonderland

Food Technology on Trial

The high visibility with which cyclamates were banned, DES
was raked over the coals, and Alar was removed from our food
supply, has produced an atmosphere in which consumers are
quick to question the safety of all food chemicals and technologies. The media have happily orchestrated these fears with
suitably hysterical headlines. The inevitable result: panic in the
pantry reigns.

This chapter takes a look at what consumers fear and then
considers the facts about various high-visibility concerns. To

153

balance this, the next chapter discusses what food experts say should be the *real* concerns about our food supply.

Consumers Express Their Fears

Several polls have tried to define what people fear most about food technology and our food supply. A 1984 Roper Poll, for example, listed six dietary items and asked consumers to state which, if any, they thought posed a threat to health. Here are the results:

Item	"Very" or "Somewhat" Concerned	"Not at all" Concerned
Salt	70%	27%
Cholesterol	65%	33%
Sugar	63%	34%
Caffeine	53%	42%
Saccharin*	36%	34%
Aspartame/NutraSweet**	30%	42%

*29 percent of respondents didn't use saccharin
**24 percent didn't use aspartame

The Sixth Annual Food Marketing Institute Survey (1988) asked one thousand shoppers which factors they considered "very important" when making their food selections. They replied: taste (88 percent), safety (83 percent), nutrition (72 percent), price (65 percent), storability (51 percent), and ease of preparation (39 percent). The surveyors also asked consumers what they thought were serious food-caused health hazards. Seventy-five percent of those surveyed said that pesticides and antibiotics were a threat to health, 61 percent answered that antibiotics and hormones in poultry and livestock concerned them, and 43 percent were concerned about irradiated food. A 1989 survey of 772 people conducted by the Gallup Organization found that over 80 percent of those surveyed were concerned about the effect of what they ate on their future health.

Let's examine these issues and several others that concern consumers.

Food Irradiation

Many people fear that irradiating food threatens public health because it reduces the nutritional value of food, introduces dangerous by-products, and even renders food radioactive. Many are also afraid that food irradiation facilities pose a nuclear threat to surrounding communities.

These fears are unjustified. Irradiated food has been studied as extensively as other food preservation processes, including canning, freezing, and dehydration. Irradiation does not destroy significant amounts of nutrients or create hazardous substances in foods. Irradiated foods do not become radioactive, and the process does not generate radioactive waste. Finally, there is no similarity between the irradiation process and nuclear weapons production when cobalt-60 (the preferred source) is used.

Over the centuries, much effort has been devoted to finding ways to preserve food and protect it from microorganisms, insects, and other pests. Drying was one of the first techniques developed. Fermenting, salting, and smoking also have long histories. Later inventions, including freezing, refrigeration, canning, and the use of preservatives and pesticides, have further increased the quality, quantity, and safety of our food supply by protecting it against contamination and spoilage.

Since 1958 food irradiation has been approved by approximately thirty-five countries, including the United States. Although this food preservation process has been successfully adopted in twenty countries, including technologically advanced countries such as Canada, France, Russia, Japan, the Netherlands, and Belgium, it has been used only for special purposes (such as for sterilizing food for patients with impaired immunity) in the United States. Here, several small but vigorous organizations have generated enough communication to persuade many prominent food companies to pledge not to use irradiated products. Opponents have also exerted similar pressure on supermarkets and state legislators. Three states have even passed laws preventing the sale of irradiated products.

Food irradiation offers many significant advantages, foremost among which is reducing the incidence of foodborne, disease-causing organisms and effectively extending the shelf life of food without adversely affecting the taste and appearance of food. Irradiation of poultry can greatly curb the incidence of salmonella, and irradiating pork can do the same for trichinosis. The U.S. Department of Agriculture estimates that the American consumer will receive approximately $2 in benefits (reduced spoilage, less illness) for each $1 spent on irradiating food.

In January 1992 a Florida-based company, Vindicator, Inc., began irradiating fruits and vegetables intended for commercial sale. A few supermarkets that have sold irradiated produce have found that consumer acceptance is high. But, so far, the poultry industry has not been willing to use irradiation.

Does BST Harm the Milk Supply?

Bovine somatotropin (BST) is a naturally occurring growth hormone composed of approximately 190 amino acids. Produced by the pituitary gland, it regulates milk production in dairy cows. Although it has been known for decades that BST supplementation makes dairy cows more productive, it could not be produced economically until recent biotechnologic breakthroughs occurred.

Synthetically produced BST, almost identical to naturally occurring BST, works within a day or so to increase milk production by 15 to 25 percent. This enables producers to respond quickly to fluctuations in the demand for milk without having to increase herd size.

Those who oppose BST are worried about two main points: first, that consumers will be drinking the hormone; second, that cows receiving BST will suffer from overstressed milk production. Neither is cause for any concern, says the FDA. After an extensive review, the FDA concluded that: "Fears about the growth hormone's effect on human health do not withstand close scrutiny." Tests show that cows receiving BST supplement have no higher BST levels in their milk than those not receiving the supplement. Whatever small amount of BST people do ingest is easily broken down, as any other protein would be, into inactive fragments in the gastrointestinal tract during digestion. In the 1950s, attempts to treat human dwarfism in children by injecting them with BST were not successful and indicated that BST has no effect on human growth. Finally, there is extensive evidence that BST does not overstress cows, harm them in any way, or interfere with their milk production.

Designer Genes

Next in the parade of "new stuff in our food supply to be scared about" is genetic engineering or biotechnology, often simply called biotech. Biotechnology is the use of living things to create new products or to change old ones. Contrary to what opponents of biotechnology would lead the public to believe, it has been around for a long time. Sometimes new plants and animals result from planned breeding, often a process of trial and error, but many occur by accident. Cattle-breeding is a time-honored example of improving stock by selectively breeding two superior animals to produce offspring with certain desired characteristics. Beefalo, on the other hand, is the result of breeding cattle with buffalo to create an entirely different animal. The tangelo is the product of crossing a tangerine with a grapefruit.

Critics of biotech don't seem concerned about tangelos. They are fighting uses of the "new biotechnology" that takes the guesswork out of selective breeding of plants and animals by allowing direct alteration of DNA, the material in living cells that carries inherited characteristics. In the new biotechnology, the gene carrying a desired trait is transferred from the DNA of one organism to that of another. This technology is not being used to produce new and different plants and animals, however. In most cases, it's used to improve on what we already have.

Billions of dollars are spent each year for insecticides and herbicides to protect plants used for food and animal feed. Biotechnology has allowed development of a number of plants, including tomatoes, potatoes, carrots, lettuce, cabbage, rice, pears, and apples that have been genetically altered to resist or tolerate herbicides, insects, and virus, and withstand drought and temperature changes. The first genetically engineered food scheduled to reach the American dinner table is a tomato that keeps longer without getting soft.

In May 1992 the government announced a policy of promoting the development of new, safe foods through biotechnology by reforming the process of regulating this industry. The policy was developed by the FDA, which has the responsibility of overseeing that foods and other products created through bio-technology pose no risk to the public. It describes the scientific basis for evaluating and ensuring the safety of new varieties of foods that are developed using any technique, including biotech. Biotechnology opponents have threatened that unless the FDA conducts a formal rulemaking procedure, they will initiate legal action to prevent genetically engineered products from being sold.

In the long run, introduction of these new products into the food supply will help lower food prices by reducing loss on the farm from insects, weeds, and viral infection, and from drought, freezing weather, and spoilage; provide foods with superior keeping qualities, appearance, flavor, and nutrition (such as reduced-fat meat or corn with increased protein); and prevent food shortages. In spite of opponents who are typically against anything they regard as not being "natural," biotech had grown to a $4 billion industry in 1991 and is projected to reach $50 billion by the year 2000.

Antibiotics in Animal Feed:
A Threat to Human Health?

Food activists have generated headlines that focus attention on the possible dangers of trace levels of antibacterial substances in cow milk, one of our most sacrosanct foods. These critics stop short of recommending that consumers, especially infants and children, discontinue milk consumption.

Antibiotics are used extensively in the raising of livestock and poultry. High doses are used to treat diseases, just as they are in human medicine. (Therapeutic levels are defined roughly as above 200 grams per ton of feed or equivalent intakes through water.) Doses below therapeutic levels are used for other pur-poses that have no parallel in current human medical practice except for low-level long-term prophylactic treatment for acne.

Antibiotics are routinely included (at levels below 100 grams/ton) in livestock and poultry feeds because they increase the rate of weight gain in growing young animals or birds. Antibiotics also increase feed efficiency (the amount of meat that can be produced from a given amount of feed) and help prevent bacterial diseases. The levels considered therapeutic vary with the drug used and the disease organism being treated, and may change over time.

Feeding antibiotics to farm animals poses a theoretical risk of increasing the prevalence of antibiotic-resistant bacteria which might cause human diseases that could not be treated successfully with the same drugs. Opponents, in fact, claim that a disease "time bomb" may soon explode as a result of more than thirty years of antibiotic use in animal agriculture. If this were true, however, smaller "time bombs" would explode first in the populations most heavily exposed to antibiotic-resistant bacteria from farm animals: the animals themselves, livestock producers, and slaughterhouse workers. The effectiveness of the drugs as animal growth promotants would also be expected to decrease. The best available evidence from extensive monitoring, however, indicates that these events have not occurred. Thus there is no reason to believe that human health is threatened by using antibiotics in animal production.

How, then, did such an unfounded attempt to undermine consumer confidence in our milk supply begin? In December 1988, the *Wall Street Journal (WSJ)* and the Nader-affiliated Center for Science in the Public Interest (CSPI) scared American consumers with two separate surveys in an article headlined, "Milk is Found Tainted with a Range of Drugs Farmers Give Cattle." The subtitle, "Residues in 38% of samples," provided little or no comfort or reassurance on the safety of our milk supply.

Unfortunately, the *WSJ* and CSPI based their alarming survey on *screening* assays and failed to perform the required *confirmatory* assay. These screening assays merely indicate that some residues of a drug class *may* be present. The word "may" is emphasized because crude screening assays often suggest the presence of a substances that cannot be confirmed by specific tests—so-called "false positive" results. The FDA then conducted a nationwide sampling and testing program with the same *screening* tests used by the *WSJ* and CSPI. The key difference was that the FDA also performed *confirmatory* assays to measure whether specific animal drug residues were present. In February 1990 the FDA concluded the following (slightly paraphrased):

A nationwide survey of milk has found no residues of any antibiotics, including sulfa drugs. These findings, based on the most current analytical methods, contradict earlier conclusions reached after publication of an unconfirmed screening test sponsored by a national newspaper.

In other words, proper assays demonstrated that our milk supply was safe and had not been contaminated by antibiotics, unauthorized drugs, or any other substance harmful to health. Professor Thomas H. Jukes, University of California at Berkeley, has furnished additional perspective (slightly paraphrased):

In the *WSJ* survey, sulfa drugs were found in the range of 5-10 milligrams per ton of milk. A dose of sulfa drugs is about 2,000 milligrams per day for an adult. To obtain such a therapeutic level, an intake of 200 tons (200,000 quarts) of milk per day would be required!

Federal and state regulatory authorities, dairy processors, and farmers continue to test millions of samples each year to ensure that our milk remains safe. Meat and poultry products also are safe. In fact, they are safer than if antibiotics were not used!

BHT and BHA

The widely used antioxidants BHT and BHA have been another target of "health food" enthusiasts who fear that these additives cause cancer.

BHT and BHA first found widespread use as antioxidants around 1947. They were added to a variety of items, such as cod-liver oil, margarine, lard, salted fish, breakfast cereals, frozen dairy products, butter, peanut oil, corn oil, safflower oil, and various other products.

Antioxidants such as BHA and BHT are added to foods to keep them safe, wholesome, and edible for longer periods of time. Although extensive studies had repeatedly confirmed the safety of BHA and BHT, these antioxidants came under closer scrutiny after the results of two isolated studies were released. One study from the early 1960s reported that BHT caused rats to bear eyeless offspring. This result was not confirmed by similar studies conducted around the world. In 1982 Japanese researchers reported that high levels of BHA produced tumors of the forestomach in rats. This finding was especially surprising because many scientists believe that the use of BHA and BHT may actually be a factor in the lower incidence and *falling* death rates of stomach cancer in the United States.

Because Americans are so quick to believe scare stories about food additives, the use of BHA and BHT was reevaluated even though the results of the Japanese studies differed greatly from those of many others. As a result of this scrutiny, these antioxidants are now restricted to current levels in foods for which they already have been approved, and testing continues.

If BHT and BHA were banned, only two alternatives would remain. Either new antioxidants will have to be found, or high-fat food products will have to be bought and eaten during their limited period of natural freshness, *and* will require constant refrigeration.

Coffee, Tea, or Methylene Chloride?

Millions of Americans feel they can't begin their day without that first eye-opening cup of coffee. However, in the last few years, both regular and decaffeinated coffee have received their share of criticism.

The "pepper-upper" in coffee and cola beverages is caffeine, a stimulant that occurs naturally in coffee, cocoa beans, tea leaves, cola nuts, and more than sixty other plants. Caffeine is actually a drug that affects the nervous system. When consumed in large amounts, it can cause nervousness, anxiety, irritability, insomnia, and disturbances in heart rate and rhythm. Caffeine also affects blood pressure, circulation of blood to the heart, and the secretion of stomach acid.

At various times caffeine has been accused of contributing to birth defects, some forms of cancer, cardiovascular disease, behavioral problems, disorders of the central nervous system, reproductive problems, and noncancerous breast lumps (fibrocystic disease) in women. Despite caffeine's effects on the central nervous system, it has not been found guilty of any of these charges, as indicated by the following statements:

• The American Cancer Society agrees with scientists who have found that there is no link established between coffee and cancer.

• Scientists reviewing the results of more than fifteen

research studies concluded that caffeine does not cause any persistent increase in blood pressure.

• No clear conclusion has been drawn about any proposed link between coffee intake and increased blood cholesterol levels. One problem may be that people with a high coffee intake appear to be more likely than light coffee drinkers to engage in unhealthy habits, such as smoking cigarettes and eating a high-fat, low-fiber diet.

• Research studies indicate that there is no established association between caffeine intake and the development of fibrocystic breast disease.

• Caffeine has never been shown to cause birth defects. (Erring on the side of caution, however, the FDA warned pregnant women to reduce their intake of caffeine or avoid it altogether.)

Health experts suggest that all Americans limit caffeine-containing products to moderate quantities. What's "moderate"? Most experts agree that the amount of caffeine in a few cups of coffee per day shouldn't present a problem except to individuals who are very sensitive to it. However, a significant percentage of people will develop caffeine-related symptoms if they drink five to six cups of coffee per day.

Concerned about caffeine, many Americans turned to decaffeinated beverages, only to be faced with new fears. Some coffee is decaffeinated by passing it through a filter containing, among other things, methylene chloride. Trouble began brewing after it was announced that rats inhaling exceedingly high concentrations of methylene chloride developed cancer. Anti-additive forces trumpeted these results and ignored more relevant studies. When laboratory animals were fed methylene chloride in amounts equaling seventy to eighty cups of decaffeinated coffee per day, there was no increase in cancer. And in studies of humans exposed to methylene chloride in the workplace for many years, there was no increase in the rate of cancer. Someone who drinks one or even a few cups of decaffeinated coffee per day shouldn't consider this risky to health. For people who continue to be concerned, however, two alternate methods of decaffeinating coffee (using ethyl acetate or water/carbon dioxide extraction methods) still have a clear record.

A New Player in the Fear-of-Additives Game

As we enter the 1990s, a new battle is brewing over food additives—this time over fat-substitutes. The following information will set the stage for this unfolding drama.

Americans eat a diet relatively high in fat. Estimates differ, but most experts agree that we consume an average of about 37 percent of our daily calories from fat, compared to a *recommended* intake of not more than 30 percent. (As high as this intake is, it is a favorable reduction from the 40 to 43 percent estimated in the mid-1980s.) Eating a high-fat diet, particularly one high in saturated fatty acids, has been linked to heart and artery disease, cancer, and, of course, overweight.

But Americans enjoy eating high-fat foods. The fat in a food often carries much of its flavor, and foods with a higher fat content have a greater satiety value, i.e., they satisfy hunger longer after you've eaten them. Giving up fat, then, means giving up much of the pleasure of eating, say many Americans.

Just as food technology supplied substitutes for sugar, it has come up with several candidates for replacing fat. Researching and developing such products is very expensive, but food companies feel that the potential market for foods that have the texture, look, and taste of high-fat products—without the liability of fat—will more than make up for their investment. As one nutritionist quipped, "it'll be bigger than Tide." But, as you might expect, battle lines were drawn even before these fat substitutes gained FDA approval. The two best-known contenders are olestra and Simplesse.

Olestra was discovered over two decades ago by research scientists at Procter & Gamble Co. They found that fatty acid esters of sugars containing six or more fatty acids weren't broken down by human fat-digesting enzymes. Since these new substances aren't broken down, they can't be absorbed by the human body. In other words, they pass through the digestive tract unchanged, contributing no calories or nutrients. The substances created by this research were first called sucrose polyesters. A specific fraction of these is called olestra.

Olestra looks and tastes like fat. To date, P&G has conducted over one hundred human and animal safety studies, all of which conclude that olestra is safe for human consumption. In 1987 P&G filed requests with the FDA to use olestra as a calorie-free fat replacement in:

• Shortenings, salad oils, and cooking oils for home use (up to 35 percent by weight of olestra).

• Commercial shortenings and oils for use in cooking or seasoning a variety of foods, in deep-fat frying, and in preparing commercial fried snacks (up to and including 75 percent by weight of olestra).

CSPI is one of the consumer groups actively working to influence the FDA to refuse approval of olestra. Citing an insufficient number of animal studies, CSPI claims that olestra is toxic and carcinogenic. As we go to press in the summer of 1992, the FDA decision is still pending, with no estimated approval date.

The NutraSweet Company's fat substitute, Simplesse, has beaten olestra to the marketplace. Unveiled in early 1988, Simplesse is described by its manufacturer as "the first and only all-natural fat substitute." It is made from a combination of water and protein (the protein is from milk, egg white, and/or whey) and provides about 1.3 calories per gram instead of the 9 calories per gram in the fat it replaces. NutraSweet doesn't plan to market Simplesse directly to the public. Instead, food manufacturers will use it to reduce fat and calories in their products "without sacrificing the desired creamy, rich taste or texture."

NutraSweet says that Simplesse isn't actually a new food additive but is simply protein from natural foods in an altered physical form (size, shape, and texture). Because of this, NutraSweet petitioned the FDA for GRAS ("generally recognized as safe") status for Simplesse. The petition was approved in March 1990. The road to approval wasn't entirely smooth, however. The FDA was unhappy that NutraSweet made public announcements about its new product before filing its petition. So far, though, the only health concerns voiced about Simplesse have to do with people who are sensitive to egg and/or milk. Consumer acceptance of Simplesse, in fact, has been quite favorable.

With the potential for affecting the dietary intake of millions of people and a multimillion- or even billion-dollar market at stake, you can be sure that the controversies over fat substitutes are just beginning.

How Much of a Concession Should Be Made for Individual Sensitivity?

Some food additives do indeed pose a special risk for highly sensitive individuals. How and how much should we legislate for these individual sensitivities? Groups like CSPI have adamantly called for the banning of such additives, including sulfites and MSG. We disagree. We believe it is preferable to warn those who are sensitive to specific additives, just as the government has done with sulfites and MSG. Here are the facts:

Sulfites

Sulfites are preservatives that have long been used in or on a wide variety of foods to reduce or prevent spoilage and discoloration during preparation, storage, and distribution. They are commonly used in fresh fruits and vegetables, processed fruits, alcoholic beverages (especially wine and beer), beverage bases, and fish and shellfish.

Sulfites have come under fire because adverse reactions surfaced as salad bars gained in popularity in the 1980s. To keep salad bar items tasting and looking fresh, sulfite sprays and dips were used more extensively. Between November 1982 and September 1987, the FDA received more than a thousand complaints regarding suspected allergic reactions to sulfites used in foods. Most cases occurred in asthmatics, a population with a much greater incidence of sulfite sensitivity. Of the approximately ten million Americans with asthma, one million are estimated to be sulfite-sensitive. Their reactions to sulfites range from hives, nausea, diarrhea, and shortness of breath, to fatal anaphylactic shock. In response to these reports, the FDA has taken the following steps:

1. As of August 1986 sulfites could no longer be used on fresh fruits and vegetables that are intended to be sold or served raw to consumers.

2. Beginning in January 1987 products containing ten parts per million (ppm) or more of sulfites had to state this fact on the label.

3. Since June 1987 pharmaceutical products containing sulfites have had to be so labeled.

4. In January 1988 the Bureau of Alcohol, Tobacco, and Firearms began requiring similar labeling for alcoholic beverages containing sulfites at a level of ten ppm or more.

5. In March 1990 the FDA banned the use of sulfites on a variety of fresh potato products (not covered by the ruling on fresh fruits and vegetables) that are served directly to customers in restaurants. This ban does not extend to the use of sulfites in dehydrated potato products.

Sulfites haven't been banned for all uses and in all products because they don't represent a risk to the vast majority of people and, in many cases, there aren't any acceptable substitutes for them in food products. The FDA's action seems to be prudent.

MSG

Monosodium glutamate, better known as MSG, is traditionally recovered from sugar beets and seaweed. MSG also can be produced synthetically in the laboratory. Put simply, MSG is the sodium salt of a common amino acid (found in all protein), which is formed in the body whenever protein is eaten. What could be more "natural"?

The ancient Orientals were probably the first to enjoy MSG's remarkable ability to enhance the flavors of their food. Although experts aren't exactly sure how MSG works, they think that it heightens the sensitivity of taste buds and increases their response to certain flavors without actually changing the food to which it has been added. One MSG advocate compared its action to "turning up the volume" on a stereo.

Another theory is that MSG enhances the flavor of food by increasing the formation of saliva. Whatever its action, many eaters feel that a little MSG, "like a little love," surely helps.

But critics say that MSG may cause some problems. First, there's "Chinese restaurant syndrome." In the late 1960s a scientist in the Washington, D.C., area began to complain of occasional lightheadedness, burning sensations, and a type of facial pressure with a tightening of facial muscles. He concluded that heavy doses of MSG used in Chinese cooking might be responsible. Subsequent studies confirmed that some individuals may indeed have a sensitivity to MSG, just as some other people may be allergic to strawberries or tomatoes. Many people who suffer migraines, for example, must avoid MSG because it can precipitate a migraine attack.

Second, there were other concerns more potentially alarming than Chinese restaurant syndrome. Dr. John W. Olney, then an associate professor of psychiatry at the Washington University School of Medicine in St. Louis, found brain damage in newborn mice and a single monkey to whom he'd administered massive injections of MSG under the skin. In another example of "bad science," these results were said to be directly applicable to babies, and a few consumer activists began to scream for the removal of MSG from baby food. Once again, the activists won, and manufacturers voluntarily removed MSG from many foods.

Whether MSG is bad or possibly even good for babies isn't really the question. What disturbed many scientists was the public's panicky reaction to the report. Some scientists asked if the source of MSG—the beet—should also be removed from the food supply on the basis of mice data, a single monkey, and a study in which the animals were injected, not fed, MSG. And what about the possible positive results of using MSG? Shouldn't these be evaluated before action is taken? For example, one study showed that under some circumstances, MSG can reduce blood cholesterol levels in man and in certain animals.

Suspicions raised about the safety of MSG have spanned two decades. In the summer of 1988, however, the Joint Expert Committee on Food Additives of the United Nations concluded that MSG doesn't represent a hazard to human health. The evidence of the more than 230 studies evaluated was so strong that the committee gave MSG its most favorable classification: an Acceptable Daily Intake that was "not specified" when it is used in foods or as a condiment.

Into the Twilight Zone: "Clinical Ecology"

When harmful substances, such as toxic chemicals, disease-causing bacteria, or viruses, enter the body, the immune system goes into action to destroy or neutralize them. However, there are times when a person's immune system identifies some harmless substance as a threat and attacks it in the same way. This is called an allergic reaction and is what happens in people who are sensitive to sulfites. By definition, an allergic reaction requires that the body's immunoglobulin E (IgE), which is part the immune system, reacts with the invading allergen and causes certain cells to pump histamine into the bloodstream. Histamine then produces the symptoms of allergy.

It's estimated that less than two percent of Americans have true food allergies. Proponents of "clinical ecology," however, say that as many as 40 percent of Americans suffer from a hypersensitivity to foods and "other environmental" factors.

"Clinical ecologists" say that any number of symptoms are triggered by a hypersensitivity to everyday foods and chemicals. Clinical ecologists include irritability, mood swings, poor memory, difficulty in concentrating, inability to think clearly, sleepiness, sneezing, running or congested nose, diarrhea, constipation, wheezing, itchy eyes and nose, muscle and joint pain, frequent urination, pounding heart, swelling of various parts of the body, and even schizophrenia and antisocial behavior on the list of symptoms that they claim can result from common stressors in the food supply and the environment. The idea that what you eat can cause antisocial or criminal behavior was even used in 1978 as the basis for the so-called "Twinkie defense" in a San Francisco murder trial.

Clinical ecologists provide a convenient answer for people suffering from multiple symptoms for which scientific practitioners can find no physical cause. For many people, simply placing the blame on a "food allergy" is preferable to identifying stress or some other hard-to-pin-down cause for their distress. After all, since clinical ecologists may label almost everything that a person comes into daily contact with as a potential "stressor," which can lead to illness, a person would have to be totally isolated not to qualify as a candidate for their services.

What can you expect if you turn to clinical ecology? If you visit a clinical ecologist, who may be an osteopathic or medical doctor, you'll probably start with such standard procedures as a physical examination, laboratory tests, and allergy tests. Then you may be asked to undergo further tests that most health professionals don't consider reliable. In provocation and neutralization tests, you'll be given various doses of substances that cause symptoms until the lowest dose that "neutralizes" the symptoms is identified. Or you may be required to follow elimination or rotation diets to try and identify the culprit foods and/or food additives.

Be aware, however, that true food allergies usually have limited symptoms—primarily skin rashes and gastrointestinal upset. Blaming chronic headaches, frequent urination, and other symptoms that may indicate a serious medical problem on food allergies can lead to delayed treatment of a real and possibly dangerous health condition.

The California Medical Association Scientific Board Task Force on Clinical Ecology, the ad hoc Committee on Environmental Hypersensitivity Disorders (established by the Minister of Health, Ontario, Canada), and the American Academy of Allergy and Immunology each conducted separate detailed and lengthy investigations of the claims and methods associated with clinical ecology. They all agreed that it is speculative and unproven.

The July 15, 1989 issue of the *Annals of Internal Medicine* contains a detailed position paper titled "Clinical Ecology." It was prepared by a nineteen-member committee of the American College of Physicians. It concludes: "Review of the clinical ecology literature provides inadequate support for the beliefs and practices of clinical ecology. . . . Diagnosis and treatments involve procedures of no proven efficacy."

Another abuse related to the diagnosis and treatment of supposed "food allergies" is cytotoxic testing. This procedure involves microscopic examination of an individual's white blood cells that have been exposed to various dried food extracts. Investigations of cytotoxic testing methods using blood samples from people with documented food allergies indicate that the test is useless. Cytotoxic testing failed to detect these true food allergies, and results from the same person differed from one day to the next.

During the early 1980s cytotoxic testing achieved notoriety when bogus "nutritionists" began offering the test in storefront clinics and through the mail. They claimed that food allergies could be responsible for virtually any health problem and that food supplements and a special diet were the answer. Fortunately, actions by federal and state enforcement agencies seem to have driven cytotoxic testing from the marketplace.

The lesson to be learned: Steer clear of practitioners who

claim that food allergies can cause a large number of diseases. This claim is false.

Now let's backtrack out of the Twilight Zone, move forward into reality, and examine real concerns about our food supply.

10

Banishing Panic from the Pantry

> "You see," he went on after a pause, "it's as
> well to be provided for *everything*. That's
> the reason the horse has all those anklets
> round his feet."
> "But what are they for?" Alice asked in a tone
> of great curiosity.
> "To guard against the bites of sharks," the
> Knight replied.
>
> —Lewis Carroll
> *Through the Looking Glass*

Is Our Food Supply Safe?

The best of scientific evidence simply cannot support the
contention that our food supply threatens our health. Eighteen
scientific groups representing more than one hundred thousand
scientists said exactly that at the conclusion of their 1989 food
safety workshop, convened by the Institute of Food Technologists' Office of Scientific Public Affairs:

> The perception that the food supply is unsafe is not sup-
> ported by scientific data. . . . Current state and federal
> legislation provides sufficient authority to protect consum-
> ers. . . . Further legislation is not required.

Surveys reveal that at least 75 percent of Americans are concerned about pesticide residues in food. This is a major misconception. Dr. Richard Adamson of the National Cancer Institute stated that "I am unaware of [any] evidence that suggests regulated and approved pesticide residues in food contribute to the toll of human cancer in the United States." Indeed, the Institute of Food Technologists also concluded that "the health effects from pesticide residues may be relatively insignificant when compared to those associated with naturally-occurring chemicals in foods."

The fourth annual FDA pesticide monitoring report (for 1990) states that more than 97 percent of the foods produced in the United States or imported from other countries either have no pesticide residues or have levels well within federally allowed limits. The report is based on testing of more than nineteen thousand produce, grain, and dairy samples from the fifty states, Puerto Rico, and ninety-two foreign countries. Of the almost nine thousand domestic foods tested, 2 percent exceeded allowed levels of residues for pesticides allowed by the Environmental Protection Agency or contained residues of pesticides not allowed for the specific food. Of the more than ten thousand imported foods that were tested for 1990, 4.3 percent were in violation of pesticide residues. Dr. Sanford Miller, a former FDA official who is now a dean at University of Texas Health Science Center at San Antonio, summed up the situation by saying, "The risk of pesticide residues to consumers is effectively zero."

Nor do cancer statistics back up the contention that Americans, or anyone else for that matter, is getting cancer because of pesticide residues, food additives, or any other aspect of modern food technology. In the first edition of this book we quoted British scientist Dr. F. J. Roe's comment that if additives were dangerous, cancer of the gastrointestinal tract should be common in highly developed countries—which is not the case. Dr. Roe's words are still true today. Let's look at death rates for cancer of the stomach across the globe:

**Table 10–1. Age-Adjusted Death Rates
(Per 100,000 People) For Stomach Cancer**

Country	1964–65		1984–86	
	Male	Female	Male	Female
United States	10.45	5.13	7.4	3.4
Canada	17.56	8.13	12.0	5.3
Australia	15.48	7.95	12.4	5.6
Denmark	21.76	13.39	14.0	7.1
Greece	16.49	10.04	14.0	7.5
Sweden	22.04	12.03	14.3	7.6
New Zealand	16.54	8.33	14.5	6.4
France	21.44	10.63	14.8	6.5
Switzerland	26.01	14.90	15.8	7.9
Norway	26.01	14.63	18.3	8.8
Scotland	25.47	14.50	19.2	10.3
Ireland	23.88	15.94	19.5	10.4
Northern Ireland	21.87	13.59	19.7	8.5
England/Wales	23.42	11.46	20.4	8.8
Netherlands	28.26	15.18	20.7	8.8
Finland	39.66	20.38	21.8	12.4
Germany (FR)	37.09	20.69	23.5	12.6
Yugoslavia	21.10	11.95	24.7	12.0*
Bulgaria	40.56	26.67	28.3	16.5
Austria	42.11	23.62	28.4	14.2
Czechoslovakia	42.74	22.59	29.3	14.4
Hungary	42.74	23.18	34.9	15.8
Poland	44.18	21.17	35.4	13.3

* 1984-85 only

Table 10–1 indicates that the United States has the lowest death rate from stomach cancer. The countries with eating habits and food preservation methods similar to those of the United States tend to have stomach cancer rates closer to ours than do countries that use substantially fewer antioxidants.

Between 1930 (when cancer statistics by site were first reported) and 1947, the U.S. and a number of similar countries reported a relatively gradual decline in the rate of stomach cancer. Many scientists believe that the increased use of BHA and BHT during this time contributed to this improvement. Animal studies support this contention: animals fed BHT and BHA have lower rates of stomach cancer than do comparison control animals.

But There Must Be Something Wrong with Our Food Supply

Should we worry about our food supply in any way? Oddly enough, issues that concern the food experts are the same issues that have plagued humans throughout history. In order of priority, the four top issues that concern food technologists are foodborne disease, malnutrition, naturally occurring environmental contaminants, and naturally occurring toxicants. Let's look at these in more detail.

Foodborne disease. The 1989 Institute of Food Technologists report says that any health risk associated with pesticide residues "is negligible and in orders of magnitude less than that of foodborne diseases such as *Salmonella* and *Shigella*." Indeed, it is estimated that up to about six million cases of food- and water-borne disease causing some nine thousand deaths may occur in the U.S. each year, at an economic cost of between one and ten billion dollars. Ironically, the back-to-nature method of food procurement and preparation that "health food" enthusiasts advocate so strongly can cause even *more* cases of foodborne disease, as we mention in chapters 3 and 4.

Malnutrition. The population of the world has been growing rapidly. Most of the world isn't preoccupied with additives and their safety, but with getting enough food to live a healthy life. Good citizens of this world can't afford to support people who preach against the use of chemical fertilizers, pesticides, and other agricultural aids. It's a simple fact that the technology that fed two billion people in the 1930s can't feed a population of five billion (and growing). In many parts of the world, starvation is already a leading cause of death, especially among young children. Intensive efforts are needed both to increase crop yield from each agricultural acre and to reduce food deterioration and wastage.

Our nation needs to move ahead in all aspects of food technology research—looking for new sources of food and new and safer additives capable of further reducing spoilage, and creating new, highly nutritious, and inexpensive food products that would be culturally acceptable in areas where supplies of food are limited. But before Americans can take this kind of rational approach to our problems, we must trust the "scientific system" and accept the fact that our current food research protocol has safety as its number one priority. In order to move toward increasing and improving our food supply through scientific knowledge, the public must have confidence in the food industry and in the regulatory agencies that govern it.

Naturally occurring toxicants. As noted in chapter 4, there are countless naturally occurring toxins that can cause disease and even death. From mushrooms to fish, many foods contain tiny amounts of these toxins. The concept that "natural" is better is simply not true and catches many "back-to-nature" people with their guard dangerously down.

Antidotes to Food Fears

How can food scares be defused? Here are some practical tips:

• Beware of science being used as a front to achieve political objectives. Peer-reviewed, mainstream science—the type worthy of reporting to readers or viewers—does not operate through media manipulations, "exclusivity agreements," or press releases. It does not use Hollywood personalities, public relations firms, or a "left wing legal activist group," as the *Wall Street Journal* has described the Natural Resources Defense Council (NRDC). Solid science is found in reputable journals where it undergoes peer review prior to publication. Such publication does not guarantee one hundred percent accuracy or that future findings will not change, but only that the report represents sound science at the time. Science advances through peer-reviewed discoveries, a point frequently overlooked by some activists, journalists, and consumers.

• Check with other reliable sources at colleges and universities. Don't rely on activists, government regulators, or industry spokespersons to be objective. If you want scientific information, call scientists. They have the expertise.

• If a purported scientific topic requires "60 Minutes," "Donahue Show," "20/20," or a partisan political group such as the NRDC to gain public attention, beware! The question is not whether the press should have done a better job in presenting NRDC's "Intolerable Risk" study, but whether the media should have reported this study at all.

• In addition to colleges and universities, registered dietitians can be an excellent source of information. Unfortunately, many poorly trained (or not trained at all!) individuals call themselves "nutritionists." Registered dietitians, on the other hand, have the initials "R.D." after their name. In states that require licensing as an additional quality control, dietitians will have the initials "R.D., L.D." after their name.

• Books, magazines, and newsletters can be another source of information, but it can be difficult to pick the roses from among the thorns. To help you choose reliable publications, the American Dietetic Association (ADA), the primary professional organization for registered and licensed dietitians in the United States, publishes a list of reputable publications. Some of the solid-science choices, plus a few of our own, are:

Reliable Books:

Fast Food Facts (Franz, 1987)
Eating on the Run (Tribole, 1987)
Jane Brody's Good Food Book (Brody, 1985)
Rating the Diets (Berland, 1986)
Jane Brody's Nutrition Book (Brody, 1987)
The New American Diet (Connor, 1986)
The New Honest Herbal: A Sensible Guide to Herbs and Related Remedies (Tyler, 1992)
Popular Nutritional Practices: Sense and Nonsense (Yetiv, 1988)
American Harvest: Regional Recipes for the Vegetarian Kitchen (Atlas, 1987)
The New Laurel's Kitchen (Robertson, 1986)
The Restaurant Companion: A Guide to Healthier Eating Out (Warshaw, 1989).
Vitamins and Minerals: Help or Harm? (Marshall, 1985)
The Health Robbers (Barrett, 1980)
Vitamins & "Health" Foods: The Great American Hustle (Herbert and Barrett, 1982)
The 100% Natural, Purely Organic, Cholesterol-Free,

Megavitamin, Low-Carbohydrate Nutrition Hoax
(Whelan and Stare, 1983)
Your Guide to Good Nutrition (Stare, Aronson, and Barrett,
1991)

Reliable Newsletters and Magazines:

Consumer Reports on Health
FDA Consumer
Harvard Health Letter
Lahey Clinic Newsletter
Living Well
Mayo Clinic Newsletter
Nutrition Forum
Tufts University Diet & Nutrition Letter
University of California, Berkeley Wellness Letter

The ADA itself offers books and cookbooks for people with special dietary needs, such as diabetics and people with food allergies. Write the American Dietetic Association for its complete publications list at 216 W. Jackson Blvd., Suite 800, Chicago, IL 60606.

On the flip side, here are some books whose covers aren't worth opening. It would be impossible to mention all the books written since the 1970s that qualify as "bad science," but here's a partial list:

Why Your Child Is Hyperactive (Feingold, 1975)
Everything You Wanted to Know about Nutrition (Ruben,
1978)
The Life Extension Weight Loss Program (Pearson and
Shaw, 1982)
Switchover! The Anti-Cancer Plan for Today's Parents and
Their Child (Long, 1984)
The Yeast Connection (Crook, 1985)

Fit for Life (Diamond and Diamond, 1985)
Dr. Berger's Immune Power Diet (Berger, 1985)
Eater's Digest and Nutrition Scoreboard (Jacobson, 1985)
Living Health (Diamond And Diamond, 1987)
Unsafe at Any Meal (Mindell, 1987)
Design Your Own Vitamin and Mineral Program
   (Lieberman, 1987).

• *Understand relevant legislation.* Perhaps the best way to
illustrate how *not* to legislate for food safety is to look carefully
at two past attempts in California, one of which was successful,
the other that failed. Proposition 65, California's so-called
"Safe Drinking Water " bill, is the perfect example of "panic in
the pantry" carried beyond Delaney to extreme and unreason-
able limits. This law, which took effect in February 1988,
requires that products as diverse as foods, gasoline, medical
devices, and alcoholic drinks carry warning labels if they
contain chemicals determined "by the state of California to
cause cancer, birth defects, and other reproductive harm." Even
before the required product labeling went into full effect,
posters at sixty-two thousand grocery stores and newspaper
advertisements provided a toll-free telephone number for consumers to call to ask about supposedly harmful substances on
sale.

What does Prop 65 really mean? Basically, it means higher
prices, fewer choices, less safe food (because additives may be
removed), and, most significantly, greater public confusion
about what is truly a threat to health.

There's a saying, *"When everything is harmful, then nothing
is harmful."* People can't spend their life worrying about the
safety of every single thing in their environment. Since, under
Prop 65, almost all products will have to be labeled as containing a possible cancer-causing substance, the result is that all
warnings will become meaningless. Warnings about cigarette

smoking, which is a well-recognized risk factor for cancer, heart disease, and a number of other serious illnesses, will have the same impact as those on hundreds of everyday foods and other products which, in reality, pose no risk at all.

Despite the confusion over Prop 65, Californians asked for more rules as they cast their November 1990 ballots. California voters faced a politically inspired ballot containing Proposition 128 ("The Big Green"), proposed by a coalition spearheaded by Assemblyman Tom Hayden and the Natural Resources Defense Council (NRDC). The initiative promised to have California lead the nation in addressing environmental concerns, including promises to save the world from the greenhouse effect, a depleted ozone layer, offshore oil spills, unsafe water, deforestation, and unsafe foods. Although these goals are worthy, the actual language of the initiative went far beyond the stated intentions and was therefore flawed.

The initiative's position on pesticides was misleading. It called for zero risk from agricultural chemicals, which would have meant restrictions of the severest sort. It would have forced communities to adhere to impossible water standards for which technologies don't even exist. It would have resulted in a 20 percent increase in utility rates; a 40 percent reduction in the supply of fresh fruits, vegetables, and field crops; and a 50 percent increase in the cost of foods for the average Californian. And it would have outlawed the use of chlorofluorocarbons (CPCs) in refrigeration and all air conditioning systems before substitutes could be developed. Fortunately, the initiative was defeated by nearly two to one.

Voters didn't care for the idea that they couldn't vote separately on some of the provisions. They realized that creating a "czar" with authority and autonomy that supersedes all levels of state government is a dangerous abuse of the traditional American system of checks and balances. It may well be that the tide is beginning to turn against the inverted priorities this initiative promoted.

• Finally, to defuse the next panic in the pantry, consider the all-important concept of relative risk. This means weighing the advantages or benefits against the disadvantages or risks. Should we accept the theoretical risk of a handful of cancers from a food preservative such as nitrates in order to prevent *certain* death and disease from not using that food chemical? This is like asking, "Should I have my ruptured appendix out and accept the minuscule risk of dying from the anesthesia, or should I accept the near-certainty of severe illness or death from that ruptured appendix?" Prudence, based on appropriate *risk-benefit analysis,* says that we should accept the smaller risks.

Some Final Thoughts

It's important to keep an open mind about all of the food substances we eat. We shouldn't just decide to condemn one type and blindly accept another. And, in thinking about health and the possibility of food and other potential environmental hazards, let's not overlook the obvious.

There are strong indications, such as Proposition 65, that the American people are paying more attention to implied or uncertain risks than they are to major and unquestioned risks to health. It is better, however, to accept the concept that nothing is "completely safe." There are only safe ways to use substances. We have a number of significant challenges to meet and many important questions to answer.

Frequent panics about this or that substance "causing cancer" or "leading to allergic reactions" do nothing but slow down the scientific search for facts. Every day, scientists all over the world come up with new findings, many of which are categorized as "preliminary." Scientific research is a slow, meticulous, repetitive process. It is counterproductive to announce "results" before they've been verified, reviewed, and confirmed. Nor is it at all helpful to the public to see a newspaper article headlined "Food and Health Experts Warn Against Bringing Home the Bacon" and reporting the views of one scientist who may or may not have reliable data to back them up. Certainly, consumers should be kept up-to-date on the results of laboratory findings, but the reports they read should be put into perspective. Unverified scare reports based on the opinion of one or two scientists (or even someone with no scientific background) should be minimized. We need responsible reporting and general public health education that provides a balanced account of the facts and helps reduce the present communication barrier between scientists and consumers.

Responsible administrators who won't feel compelled to act on the basis of rumor are key to controlling panic. In 1973 the President's Science Advisory Committee concluded:

> Where knowledge is so inadequate as to make the reality of a possible threat quite tenuous, the proper response is to seek more knowledge, not either to take drastic action or to do nothing.

We need food legislation that allows us to judge what we eat not by the labels "natural" or "artificial" or because animals fed unrealistic quantities of substances get tumors. Useful laws would allow for advances in scientific knowledge and would assess foods based on a combination of relevant data: benefits, safety, acceptability, and ill-effects. Indeed, the President's Science Advisory Committee recommended:

> The growing and changing nature of scientific knowledge demands flexibility in regulatory procedures—not rigidity.

Laws, regulatory structures, and styles of administrative action all need to be adapted to a continuing growth and change in knowledge.

To state it yet another way, America needs food laws that will permit us to enter our pantries with a feeling of confidence and a sense of assurance that what we find there is safe. *And* Americans should be able to know, without a doubt, that what has been removed was banned for legitimate, scientific reasons, not because our laws couldn't keep up with advances in technology and scientific understanding.

We must struggle harder against the harmful effects of food faddism, "health food" charlatans, and rumors about the hazards of specific foods. At best, food fads are luxuries that are inconsistent with the realities of worldwide food shortage and rising food costs. At worst, these fads steal scarce financial resources and pose unnecessary health risks.

Today most Americans can maintain a pantry stocked with food that is wholesome, nutritious, safe, varied, affordable, and tasty. Let's safeguard our good fortune by dealing calmly and rationally with new facts about food technology.

Selected References

Additive-free diet doesn't correct behavioral problems. *American Family Physician* 20:145, 1979.

Additives, apples, etc. (Editorial). *American Family Physician* 18:66, 1978.

AMA Council on Scientific Affairs. Aspartame: Review of safety issues. *Journal of the American Medical Association* 254:400, 1985.

——— Saccharin: Review of safety issues. *Journal of the American Medical Association* 254: 2622, 1985.

American Cancer Society. Cancer facts & figures–1990.

Americans for Safe Food. *Guess What's Coming to Dinner.* Washington, D.C., Center for Science in the Public Interest, 1987.

Ames, B.N., et al. Ranking possible carcinogenic hazards. *Science* 236:271, 1987

Anderson, J.A., et al: Position statement on clinical ecology. *Journal of Allergy Clinical Immunology* 78: 269, 1986.

Annino, L., et al. Non-prescription medications from health food stores: A potential source of serious illness. *Connecticut Medicine* 35:428, 1971.

Arriving at judgments on health hazards. *Federation Proceedings* 36:2544, 1977.

Aspartame: good news. *Newsweek*, Nov. 16, 1987.

Attorney general vs. phony health food claims. *Changing Times,* May 1973.

Barrett, S. Fighting quackery: A quick reference guide. *Postgraduate Medicine* 81:13, 1987.

——— Health or hype?—A report on United Sciences of America. New York, American Council on Science and Health, 1987.

——— The multilevel mirage. *Priorities,* Summer 1991.

——— Proposed labeling rules stir controversy. *Nutrition Forum,* Jan./Feb. 1992.

——— Should nutritionists be licensed? *Postgraduate Medicine* 79:11, 1986.

——— Unproven "allergies": an epidemic of nonsense. *Nutrition Today* 24(2):6, 1989.

Beloian, A. Nutrition labels: A great leap forward. *FDA Consumer,* Sept. 1973.

Bernarde, M.A. *The Chemicals We Eat.* New York, American Heritage Press, 1971.

Bernhardt, C.A. Olestra: A non-caloric fat replacement. *Food Technology International—Europe,* 1988.

Bitter sweetener. *Time,* Aug. 26, 1974.

Bleiberg, R.M. Cyclamate ban: It has cost producers and consumers dear. *Barron's,* Oct. 7, 1974.

Blix, G. Development and features of nutrition fallacies in Sweden. In (G. Blix, ed.) *Food Cultism and Nutrition Quackery.* Uppsala, The Swedish National Foundation (printed by Almquist and Wiksells), 1970.

Borchert, P., et al. The metabolism of naturally occurring hepatocarcinogen safrole. *Cancer Research* 33:575, 1973.

Borlaug, N.E. In *Proceedings of the Western Hemisphere Nutrition Congress.* Chicago, American Medical Association, 1972.

Borman, S.A. Origins of risk assessment. *Analytical Chemistry*, December 1983.

Bove, F.J. *The Story of Ergot*. New York, S. Karger, 1970.

Bowerman, S.J.A., and Harrill, I. Nutrient consumption of individuals taking or not taking nutrient supplements. *Journal of the American Dietetic Association* 83:298, 1983.

Bradstock, M.K., et al. Evaluation of reactions to food additives: the aspartame experience. *American Journal of Clinical Nutrition* 43:464, 1986.

Brody, J.E. Carcinogens: unchecked. They threaten an epidemic. *New York Times*, Oct. 6, 1974.

———— Group of scientists warns against ban on cancer-causing food additives. *New York Times*, Jan. 21, 1973.

———— Vitamin E claims held misleading: Academy of Sciences panel warns public on 'cures.' *New York Times*, Sept. 12, 1973.

Brown, R.G. Possible problems of large intakes of ascorbic acid. *Journal of the American Medical Association* 224:1529, 1973.

Bruch, H. The allure of food cults and nutrition quackery. *Nutrition Reviews*, July 1974, (special supplement)

Butz, E.L. This Week. *New Jersey Farm Bureau*, July 10, 1971.

Chemicals and Health. Report of the Panel on Chemicals and Health of the President's Science Advisory Committee, Sept. 1973.

Christiansen, L., et al. Effect of nitrite and nitrate on toxin production. *Applied Microbiology* 25:357, 1973.

'Citizen enforcers.' The *Wall Street Journal*. June 15. 1987.

Citizens' Commission on Science, Law and the Food Supply: A report on current ethical considerations in the determination of acceptable risk with regard to food and food additives, Jan. 28, 1974.

Colloway, D. Are health foods worth it? *McCalls,* Oct. 1971.

Congress to the rescue. *Time,* May 20, 1985.

Coon, J. Natural food toxicants: A perspective. *Nutrition Reviews* 11:321, 1974.

—— The Delaney Clause. *Preventive Medicine* 2:150, 1973.

Cyclamate: a reappraisal. *Science News,* June 15, 1985.

Cyclamates: Hearing before the ad hoc Subcommittee of the Committee on the Judiciary, United States Senate. Ninety-second Congress, Second Session on H.R. 13366, Sept. 7, 8, 1972, Washington, D.C., United States Government Printing Office, 1972.

Damo, G.E. Primer on food additives. Department of Health, Education, and Welfare Publication 74-2002, 1973.

Deutsch, R. *The Family Guide to Better Food and Better Health.* Creative Home Library, 1971.

—— Food fads: fantasy and fact. In *Food and Fitness*, Blue Cross Association, 1973.

—— *The New Nuts Among the Berries.* Palo Alto, California, Bull Publishing Company, 1977.

—— Where you should be shopping for your family. *Nutrition Reviews*, July 1974 (special supplement).

Dougherty, P.H. Advertising: on health cereals. *New York Times*, Jan. 30, 1974.

Edwards, C.E. Testimony before the Subcommittee on Intergovernmental Relations, House Committee on Government Operations, Washington, D.C., March 16, 1971.

Egeberg, R.O., et al. Report to the Secretary of HEW from the Medical Advisory Group on Cyclamates. *Journal of the American Medical Association* 211:1358, 1970.

Epstein, S. The Delaney Amendment. *Preventive Medicine* 2:140, 1973.

Esajian, J. California's Proposition 65: A sop to environmentalists? *Medical Tribune*, March 31, 1988.

Estimated sales of over-the-counter internal medications. *FDA Consumer*, Oct. 1986.

Evans, I., et al. The possible human hazard of the naturally occurring bracken carcinogen. *The Biochemistry Journal* 124:28, 1971.

Fairweather, F.A. Food additives and cancer. *Proceedings of the Nutrition Society* 40:21, 1981.

Fat substitutes on the horizon. *Calorie Control Commentary*, Spring 1988.

FDA information sheets on additives, dietary supplements, etc. undated (obtained in 1988).

Finch, R. HEW Press Release, Oct. 18, 1969.

Five color additives approved. *FDA Consumer,* Sept. 1986.

Food additives: An industry view. *FDA Consumer*, Dec. 1977/ Jan. 1978.

Food Chemical News, 1970–1974, 1987–1988.

Food safety a growing concern. *FDA Consumer,* Sept. 1988.

Freedman, A.M. As 'fresh refrigerated' foods gain favor, concerns about their safety rise. *The Wall Street Journal*, March 11, 1988.

Fuller, J.G. *The Day of St. Anthony's Fire.* New York, Macmillan, 1968.

Gold, G. Egg substitute is rated on nutrition. *New York Times*, March 7, 1974.

Green, R.C. Nutmeg poisoning. *Virginia Medical Monograph* 86:586, 1959.

Grigg, W. Quackery: It costs more than money. *FDA Consumer*, July/Aug. 1988.

Guldager, B. et al. EDTA treatment of intermittent claudication—a double blind, placebo-controlled study. *Journal of Internal Medicine* 231:261–267, 1992.

Health survey: The results. *New Age Journal*, Sept./Oct. 1987.

Hecht, A. DES: the drug with unexpected legacies. *FDA Consumer*, May 1979.

—— DES keeps cropping up. *FDA Consumer*, July/Aug. 1983.

—— DES update. *FDA Consumer*, April 1986.

—— and Willis, J. Sulfites: Preservatives that can go wrong. *FDA Consumer*, Sept. 1983.

Hegsted, D. and Ausman, L. Sole foods and some not so scientific experiments. *Nutrition Today*, Nov./Dec. 1973.

Henderson, L.M. Programs to combat nutritional quackery. *Nutritional Reviews*, July 1974 (special supplement).

Herbert, V. The vitamin craze. *Archives of Internal Medicine* 140:173, 1980.

Herbst, A., et al. Adenocarcinoma of the vagina: Association of maternal stilbestrol therapy with tumor appearance in young women. *New England Journal of Medicine* 284:878, 1971.

Holbrook, S. *The Golden Age of Quackery*. New York, Macmillan, 1959.

Hopkins, H. Regulating vitamins and minerals. *FDA Consumer*, July/Aug. 1976.

Hunter, B.T. Sulfites: Preserving food at a price. *Consumers' Research*, June 1985.

Hutt, P.B. Letter to Senators Gaylord Nelson, George McGovern, Alan Cranston and Representatives Michael Harrington and Bob Eckhardt. Rockville, Md., July 9, 1973.

—— Unpublished manuscript, April 13, 1972.

Inhorn, S.L. and Meisner, L.F. Irresponsibility of the cyclamate ban. *Science* 167:1436, 1970.

Institute of Food Technologists' Expert Panel on Food Safety and Nutrition. Sweeteners: Nutritive and nonnutritive. *Contemporary Nutrition* 12(9), 1987.

W.F. Janssen. The squad that ate poison. *FDA Consumer*, Dec.

1981/Jan. 1982.

Johnson, A. and Wolfe, S. Cancer prevention and the Delaney Clause. Health Research Group, Washington, D.C., undated.

Jukes, T.H. Estrogens in beefsteaks. *Journal of the American Medical Association* 229:14, 1974.

—— The Delaney 'anti-cancer' clause. *Preventive Medicine* 2:133, 1973.

—— Scientific agriculture at the crossroads. *Nutrition Today* 8:31, 1973.

—— Fact and fancy in nutrition and food science. *Journal of the American Dietetic Association* 59:203, 1971.

Lang, S. Future food. *Vogue*, Oct. 1985.

Lave, L.B. Health and safety risk analyses: Information for better decisions. *Science* 236:291, 1987.

Lawler, P.F. *Sweet Talk*. Washington, D.C., The Media Institute, 1986.

C.W. Lecos. Caffeine jitters: some safety questions remain. *FDA Consumer*, Dec. 1987/Jan. 1988.

—— The growing use of irradiation to preserve food *FDA Consumer*, July/Aug. 1986.

—— 'An order of fries—Hold the sulfites.' *FDA Consumer*, March 1988.

—— Reacting to sulfites. *FDA Consumer*, Dec. 1985/Jan. 1986.

—— Sulfites: FDA limits uses, broadens labeling. *FDA Consumer*, Oct. 1986.

—— Sweetness minus calories = controversy. *FDA Consumer*, Feb. 1985.

Little, L.C. and MacKinney, G. The color of foods. *World Review of Nutrition and Dietetics* 14:59, 1972.

Mansfield, L.E. Food allergy and headache. *Postgraduate Medicine* 63:46, 1988.

Manufacturing Chemists Association. *Food Additives: Every-*

day Facts. Washington, D.C., 1973.

———— *Food Additives: Who Needs Them?* Washington, D.C., 1974.

Marshall, C.W. *Vitamins and Minerals: Help or Harm?* Philadelphia, George F. Stickley Company, 1985.

Mayer, J. The Delaney Clause: A sleeping watchdog. *New York Daily News*, Oct. 16, 1974.

———— *United Sates Nutrition Policies in the Seventies*. San Francisco, W.H. Freeman and Company, 1973.

Meister, K.M. Do health food stores give sound nutrition advice? *ACSH News and Views*, May/June 1983.

Miller, H.I. and Ackerman, S.J. Perspective on food biotechnology. *FDA Consumer*, March 1990.

Modeland, V. America's food safety team: A look at the lineup. *FDA Consumer*, July/Aug. 1988.

Mother nature and her chemicals join us for Thanksgiving dinner (press release). American Council on Science and Health, Nov. 20, 1987.

National Academy of Sciences, Washington, D.C. *Toxicants Occurring Naturally in Foods*, 1973.

NCAHF Newsletter (National Council Against Health Fraud, Inc.), 1985–1988.

Newberne, P.M. and Conner, M.W. Food additives and contaminants. *Cancer* 58:1851, 1986.

No evidence of MSG link to 'Chinese restaurant syndrome' concludes U.N. expert committee. News release from the Glutamate Association, June 20, 1988.

Olestra information provided by Procter & Gamble.

On regulating safety . . . and quality. *FDA Consumer*, April 1979.

Organic foods, a scientific status summary by the Institute of Food Technologists' Expert Panel on Food Safety and Nutrition and the Committee on Public Information. *Food Tech-*

nology, January 1974.

Patulin, a carcinogenic myotoxin found in cider. *Nutrition Reviews* 32:55, 1974.

Pauling, L. Ascorbic acid and the common cold. *American Journal of Clinical Nutrition* 24:1294, 1971.

Power failure for the 'immune power' diet. *Consumer Reports*, February 1986.

Recommendations concerning supplement usage. ADA Statement, *Journal of the American Dietetic Association* 87:1342, 1987.

Retired Persons Services, Inc. Activitamins and the protector vitamins. *NAD Case Report*, Council of Better Business Bureaus, 1988.

Ribon, A. and Joshi, S. Is there any relationship between food additives and hyperkinesis? *Annals of Allergy* 48:275, 1982.

Rodericks, J.V. Hazards from nature: Aflatoxins. *FDA Consumer*, May 1978.

Russell, M. and Gruber, M. Risk assessment in environmental policy-making. *Science* 236:286, 1987.

Saffiotti, U. Comments on the scientific basis for the Delaney Clause. *Preventive Medicine* 2:125, 1973.

Salt heads health concerns. *FDA Consumer*, Dec. 1984/Jan. 1985.

Schiffman, S.S., et al. Aspartame and susceptibility to headache. *New England Journal of Medicine* 317:1181, 1987.

Segal, M. Too many drinks spiked with urethane. *FDA Consumer*, April 1988.

Shell, E.R. Sweetness and health. *The Atlantic*, August 1985.

Simplesse information supplied by the NutraSweet Company.

P. Slovic: Perception of risk. *Science* 236:280, 1987.

Some not-so-bad news on caffeine. *FDA Consumer*, May 1987.

Special concerns over 'quick-fix' foods. *FDA Consumer*, July/Aug. 1988.

Stare, F.J. Combating misinformation: A continuing challenge to health professionals. *Nutrition Today* 27(3):43–46, 1992.

—— et al. "Health foods: Definitions and nutrient values. *Journal of Nutrition Education* 4:94–97, 1972.

—— How unfortunate. *Nutrition Today* 21(5):12–15, 1986.

—— and Whelan, E.M. Our foods are safe. *Mayo Clinic Proceedings* 65:1631–1632, 1990.

Stewart, M.L., et al. Vitamin/mineral supplement use: A telephone survey of adults in the United States. *Journal of the American Dietetic Association* 85:1585, 1985.

Sun, M. Food dyes fuel debate over Delaney. *Science* 229:739, 1985.

Thompson, R.C. Food allergies: Separating fact from 'hype.' *FDA Consumer*, June 1986.

—— Purifying food via irradiation. *FDA Consumer*, October 1981.

Thomsen, P.A., et al. Adolescents' beliefs about and reasons for using vitamin/mineral supplements. *Journal of the American Dietetic Association* 87:1063, 1987.

Toufexis, A. Food fight over gamma rays. *Time*, Sept. 22, 1986.

The vitamin pushers. *Consumer Reports*, March 1986.

Vitamins, minerals and the FDA. *FDA Consumer*, DHEW Publication 74-2001, 1973.

Wender, E.H. The food additive-free diet in the treatment of behavior disorders. *Journal of Developmental and Behavioral Pediatrics* 7:35, 1986.

Whelan, E.M. Can you separate food fads from facts? *Glamour*, June 1974.

—— Fads vs. facts: What's your food IQ? *Reader's Digest*, March 1975.

—— How sweet it isn't. *National Review*, Jan. 4, 1974.

—— and Stare, F.J. Nutrition. *Journal of the American Medical Association* 263:2661–2663, 1990.

Index